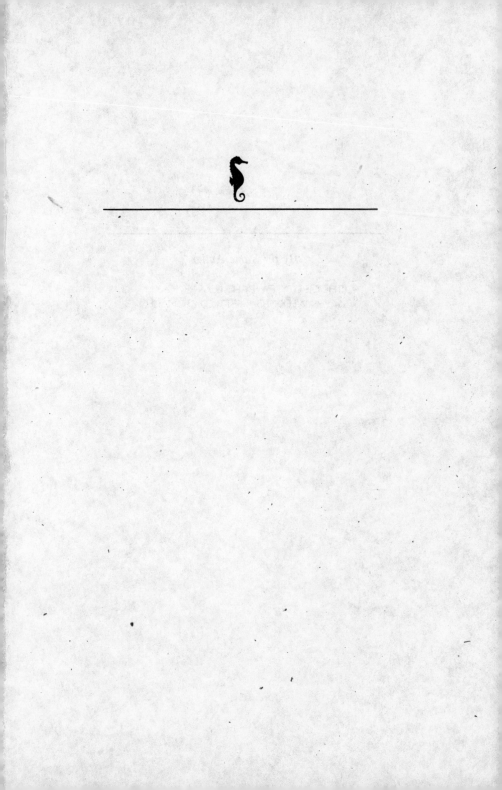

TIRED
ALL THE TIME

*How to Regain Your
Lost Energy*

▼

RONALD L. HOFFMAN, M.D.

Poseidon Press
New York • London • Toronto • Sydney • Tokyo • Singapore

POSEIDON PRESS

Simon & Schuster Building
Rockefeller Center
1230 Avenue of the Americas
New York, New York 10020

Designed by Liney Li
Manufactured in the United States of America

ISBN: 0-671-78139-1

ACKNOWLEDGMENTS

▼

My special gratitude to Jill Neimark for her invaluable help with this book; to Elaine Pfefferblit, my editor, for her encouragement with this and other book projects; to the innumerable patients who have opened their lives to me, and whose courage and determination in the face of overwhelming hardship have been a beacon to me; to the dedicated staff of the Hoffman Center, a living laboratory for the principles embodied in this book; and to my wife, Helen, who has shared my vision and provided loving support for seventeen years.

ACKNOWLEDGMENTS

I dedicate this book to the memory of Carlton Fredericks, nutrition pioneer, researcher, author, lecturer, and beloved radio personality. His work opened up vast intellectual horizons for me, and I deeply prize his legacy. I thank his wife, Betty, too, for the opportunity to have her in my life and to love her.

CONTENTS

▼

1

HOW DID WE GET SO TIRED?

▼

It is part of the cure to wish to be cured.
—Seneca

Too many Americans feel tired—all the time. If you are like many of my patients, sometimes you feel you're barely functioning: you are exhausted, dragged out, and run down. You have to push yourself through the day, struggle through your exercise classes, rouse yourself to drive your children to their lessons. You used to sink into a warm, clean bed with a feeling of blissful relief; now you're so tired you hardly have time to notice when you finally crawl into bed after a busy day. And when you wake in the morning you feel heavy and achy, far from refreshed. At 3 P.M. you sometimes lay your weary head on your desk for a moment's rest. Even on the weekends, when you catch up on sleep, you feel listless.

You're not alone. Americans make a shocking 500 million office visits to doctors every year to complain about generalized fatigue. If the number-one complaint of patients is flu and colds, tiredness is number two. Nearly half of the visitors to my own clinic come because of a mysterious, nonspecific ailment that seems to be ruining their lives: exhaustion. Fatigue has come to be seen as a genuine illness in itself. In a random survey of the U.S. population six years ago, one out of every five women and one out of every six men complained of constant fatigue. And a study of 1,200 patients at an army hospital in San Antonio found that 28 percent of women and 19 percent of men said fatigue was a major problem.

In fact, so many Americans are feeling drained that the Centers for Disease Control (CDC) in Atlanta have formally acknowledged and begun to study a "new" disease called CFS, which stands for chronic fatigue syndrome. It's an epidemic, according to many experts, and its main presenting symptom is bone-deep weariness. "I'm too tired to turn the page of a book," said one patient.

CFS is indeed a significant cause of chronic fatigue—but it is a complex disease resulting from a delicate interplay of many factors, and it is far from the only form of our modern plague of tiredness. Many doctors are hunting for a "single" cause of CFS—a virulent, unknown virus—but they probably won't find it. The route to CFS may be a circuitous one. But CFS tells us unequivocally that tiredness is rampant—and that American doctors are worried about it.

They're worried because they can't find the cause. I'm not surprised. Most doctors, unfortunately, take a conventional bull's-eye approach to fatigue: they attempt to rule out serious diseases that can be detected by blood tests, or techniques like X rays or colonoscopy. They're guided in that approach by the medical model, which seeks to harvest from the vast procession of patients a few "real" diseases, such as leukemia, brain tumors, or colitis. Although this rule-it-out approach safeguards patients who are suffering from serious diseases, it also does a great disservice to the vast majority, who are suffering from fatigue due to less obvious causes. Though doctors may content themselves with reassuring patients that they are not in immediate danger of dying, that doesn't pour energy back into an exhausted patient's life.

Another unfortunate error doctors sometimes make is to assume that fatigue not obviously physical in origin must be psychological. There's a false dichotomy in that belief, which pervades all areas of medicine: that whatever is not on the medical map is in the province of psychology.

There's another possibility: that the fatigue a patient is suffering is in the *terra incognita* of undiscovered knowledge about the body. We need to explore that *terra incognita*.

In fact, in most doctors' vocabulary, fatigue is a wastebasket diagnosis, one that is given when there is no organic, correctable cause of malaise. *Fatigue* is such a pejorative term—astonishingly, still so scoffed at by many doctors that the patient-support organization for CFS went through a long, heated debate about keeping the word *fatigue* in their name. They felt the word trivialized a potent disease process, but that bone-deep tiredness was a hallmark of the disease.

"Learn to live with your fatigue" is the advice many of my patients hear. By the time they come to me they seem almost to be auditioning for illnesses—not because they are hypochondriacs, but because they hope to find a name for their chronic tiredness so that their doctor will take it seriously. Too often they've been dismissed with the answer: "It's not serious. It's not a fatal disease."

And yet fatigue can be devastating. It saps the joy from life. I take it very seriously. I specialize in fatigue. I work as a physician problem solver, handling the chronic illnesses that often seem to have no cause and fall through the interstices of medicine. I have lectured frequently at CFS gatherings, have been interviewed by local and national media on chronic fatigue, and attend many conferences each year on everything from sleep disorders to nutrition. I was in the vanguard of innovative physicians who recognized the existence of CFS, long before the CDC recognized that there was something afoot. I'm also one of the few physicians who are fellows of both the American College for Advancement in Medicine (which focuses on nutrition, vitamins, and innovative therapies like chelation to combat degenerative diseases) and the American Academy of Environmental Medicine (which is the foremost organization in the country examining the link between environment and illness, from allergies to chemical sensitivities).

I also consider myself a compulsive information cruncher. Weekly I plow through at least a dozen medical journals, both conventional and alternative. On my desk right now are *The New England Journal of Medicine, The American Journal of Clinical Nutrition,* and a monograph on a new cholesterol-lowering herb. The moniker bestowed on me by the newspaper *New York Native* was "New York's Top Chronic Fatigue Doctor."

With all this experience under my belt, I truly believe that every one of you reading this book can treat—and conquer—your tiredness. In my private practice, I've successfully treated innumerable cases of fatigue. The reason I've been successful is that I approach each person as a medical mystery, and I fully examine and test for the most common fatigue factors that create what I think of as a "fatigue wheel." It's the kind of pie chart you're familiar with from news reports.

No two people's fatigue wheels are exactly alike. You may have succumbed to a single overriding cause of fatigue, or you may suffer from several. Even if there are many causes for your fatigue, two or three are probably going to be the most important sources of your

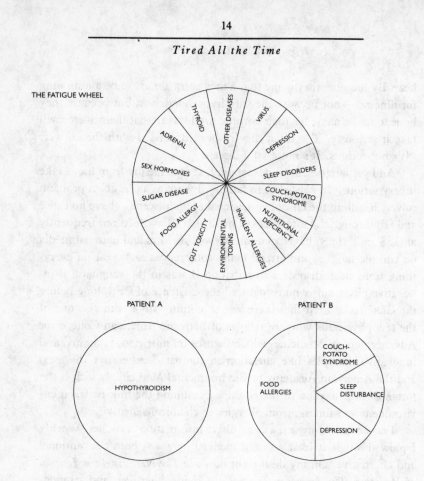

THE FATIGUE WHEEL

(Wheel labels, clockwise:) OTHER DISEASES, VIRUS, DEPRESSION, SLEEP DISORDERS, COUCH-POTATO SYNDROME, NUTRITIONAL DEFICIENCY, INHALENT ALLERGIES, ENVIRONMENTAL TOXINS, GUT TOXICITY, FOOD ALLERGY, SUGAR DISEASE, SEX HORMONES, ADRENAL, THYROID

PATIENT A

HYPOTHYROIDISM

PATIENT B

COUCH-POTATO SYNDROME

FOOD ALLERGIES

SLEEP DISTURBANCE

DEPRESSION

chronic exhaustion. One patient may have a huge pie slice called hypothyroidism—and thyroid medication may bring her back to buoyant energy. Another patient may be suffering from food allergies, couch-potato syndrome, a lack of sleep, and depression after his divorce. His four pie slices may all be important, but we may discover that identifying and treating his lifelong food allergies are the final key to health.

When I work with patients, I usually sit down with paper and pencil and make a pie chart with about twelve slices. Then I take inventory of their fatigue in response to my questions. They find that some possible causes of fatigue have no bearing on their case, while others seem tailor-made for them. You can create your own fatigue wheel as you read through this book, which contains many quizzes and questionnaires to help you determine what the causes of your fatigue might be.

Sometimes the answer is amazingly simple, and I feel like a character in the famous Edgar Allan Poe story "The Purloined Letter." An important letter has been stolen—and nobody can find it, because it is sitting on the desk in clear sight of all. That was the case with a young woman who came to me after the stillbirth of her first baby. She felt moody, sad, sluggish, and tired, and attributed her debilitating fatigue to grief over the loss of her child. So did her obstetrician.

However, there was an obvious clue to her tiredness that everyone had overlooked. Because she had begun to gain extra weight after the pregnancy, I ran some basic hormone tests and discovered that she was profoundly low in thyroid hormone. On her next visit, I asked her some simple questions, and found that she had every classic symptom of hypothyroidism: her skin was dry, her hair had thinned, she was eating the same amount as before and gaining weight, and she was constipated, cold, tired, and depressed. More amazing, both her mother and sister were hypothyroid, but she hadn't thought to mention it. As soon as she started taking low-dose thyroid hormone, she began to lose weight and her moods improved; a year later she gave birth to a healthy baby.

Although her case was startlingly "easy," I sometimes feel terribly frustrated by an initial inability to help a victim of extreme fatigue. Nevertheless, the one lesson I've learned in this practice is to keep plugging away. It may seem like dumb optimism, but I have many times seen patients who suddenly get better after a long trial of one therapy or another.

One such patient, an Orthodox Jew and father of five, came in with his seventeen-year-old daughter. "She's feeling so sick, doctor," he said. "She used to be an A student and now her grades are poor. She has headaches and she's always tired." Blood tests revealed nothing special. Her thyroid was normal. Her digestion was normal. She had a loving family and lots of friends and no particular reason to be depressed. I was stumped. Then, during one visit, he offhandedly mentioned that his whole family seemed to have a virus. "Everybody in my family is sick. We all feel cranky. The only one who feels good is my son who is off at Yeshiva."

It turned out there had been a fire in the home, and the fire department had soaked one wall with hundreds of gallons of water. Soon after, the wall became discolored—and they began to get tired and feel sick. This prompted me to think of molds. But they'd never connected indoor molds to their fatigue. The proverbial light bulb went on in my head, and I immediately walked father and daughter over to our allergy lab, where we gave them some special mold plates and told them to open these plates in their home. Sure enough, the plates came back with sky-high scores for a few species of mold.

Armed with this new clue, my patient packed his family off to upstate New York for the summer, and everyone began to feel better. On his return, he took a sledgehammer to the wall and, in a calculated fury, knocked it all down. As the plaster rained on his head, he discovered it was matted thickly with mold. He hauled fifty bags of rubble and dank, moldy plaster out into the street and was sick for a week afterward. But since then, his family's health has "magically" improved.

The reason I know you can conquer your fatigue is that I conquered mine. In the process, I learned some surprising secrets about energy—secrets that fly in the face of some of our conventional wisdom.

When I was in my teens and early twenties, I fell into the typical pattern of college students at major universities. I was a nocturnal animal, pulling all-nighters before exams with frequent trips to the coffee and snack machines. I prided myself on my beer-swilling prowess, and was a resolute couch potato. My idea of recreation was to open a can of beer while smoking a pack of Pall Malls and watching reruns of *Casablanca*. I made my A's, but I dragged through every morning, had a tendency to crash in mid-afternoon, and almost never felt energized and ebullient.

Not surprisingly, I rarely exercised. I didn't think my body was designed for exercise—I took to heart my mother's childhood warning "Don't get overheated," and used to joke with my friends that in medieval Europe the prelude to pneumonia and death was "the Sweat." I remember the day it all began to change.

It was my final year of college. I was watching the Three Stooges on television and smoking a cigarette on a Sunday morning when my roommate came striding by in athletic shorts. "It's a beautiful spring day," he said. "Want to take a run in the park?" Uncharacteristically, I stubbed out my cigarette and accepted the challenge. After just a quarter mile I felt wrenching chest pain. "This is no way to feel at the age of twenty-one," I thought. That year, I stopped smoking. I improved my diet. I began to run daily.

Today, at forty, I'm a different man. My working hours often stretch from eight in the morning to eight or nine at night. I travel to conferences, attend meetings, write books and articles, and train for triathlons and marathons. Often at 10 P.M., when my energy is flagging and I can start thinking of the delicious pleasures of sleep, I hop on the StairMaster at home and start to exercise. Half an hour later I'm carried on an astonishing wave of fresh energy that lasts for another hour or two as I review difficult cases or read the latest nutrition news in scientific journals.

I have learned some cardinal secrets to beating fatigue, which I'll expand on in this book. The first and most important is this: *Energy begets energy*. Have you ever known people who seem to rise refreshed in the morning, and to attack their day with a gusto that seems to increase with each passing hour? They appear to be made of different stuff from the ordinary person. But they're not. People who put out tremendous energy are energized by their very activity. Physical activity oxygenates all parts of the body, including the brain. It enhances circulation, and increases the metabolism. The result? Energy.

Once you begin to correct the flaws in your lifestyle, diet, and physiology that may be contributing to your fatigue, you will find that your energy begins to improve *dramatically*.

Another cardinal secret: *Life is not a steady downhill process*. Doctors are taught to accept the premise that lack of vitality, when it occurs, is a natural consequence of aging. While this is ultimately true, your energy quotient can be sustained at high levels well through middle age and into your senior years. Your body does not have to become steadily less efficient and energetic as you get older. We do not all resemble dying dwarf stars, fading inevitably from a high-energy state to a low-energy state.

In treating fatigue, I've repeatedly come across yet another secret: *Efforts to conserve energy can leave you more exhausted*. It sounds like a paradox, doesn't it? Most people think resting a lot will cure their fatigue—yet it often makes it worse. It seems that people who say, "I know the grocery is only six blocks away, but I'm so tired I'll call them up and have them deliver," are the most fatigued. If you use a mechanistic model and regard your body as a car, and your food as high-octane gasoline, you'll never fully understand the nature of fatigue in humans. I've discovered that when I'm tired, sleep isn't always the answer.

Another secret? *Stimulants may give you a short-term boost, but over the long run they can deplete you.* I'll never forget the perfect proof of this. A few years ago an amazing study showed up in a journal called *The Archives of Internal Medicine.* Patients came to their doctors suffering from terrible exhaustion. It turned out they were suffering from "caffeinism." They drank up to thirty cups of coffee a day and were absolutely depleted and listless. I once had a patient like that—he was the tiredest person I ever saw, dark circles under his eyes, listless, pale, with an exhausted, foot-dragging gait. Guzzling gallons of coffee daily had left him totally wired—but ultimately depleted. His body had no reserves left.

Another fact of fatigue is this: *Fatigue can sometimes be contagious*—just like a yawn. Sometimes, examining a patient who is having great difficulty coming to grips with his illness, who is feeling terribly defeated and pessimistic, and whose problem does not respond well to nutritional or lifestyle modifications, I find myself overcome by a draining ennui. Ten minutes later I may be sitting with another patient for whom I have had a sudden insight or solution, and I feel energized and stimulated.

When doctors say, "It's all in your head," or "Take a vacation," they may sometimes be right—and yet they underestimate how tired the body can get when the mind is depressed. I remember one patient who came in exhausted—he slumped in the chair, and his head drooped forward like a wilted flower. He complained of always being tired, every minute of the day. I was concerned. I ordered thyroid tests on him and a few weeks later he came back. His first words were, "I've been on jury duty the past two weeks, and I've discovered what was wrong with me." I uttered some sympathetic words on the tedium of two weeks in court, when he burst out, "No, no, jury duty was great! I was out of the office, and this wonderful drama was unfolding in front of me. Suddenly I felt fine! It's my *job* that's wrong. I hate my job." I hear this kind of "Aha!" discovery from my patients quite frequently. Someone will come to me and say, "You know, when I was sailboarding, scuba diving, and playing tennis at Club Med, I didn't feel fatigued at all."

I've worked hard to combat my patients' fatigue in the last decade. Whether they've ended up tearing down moldy walls, correcting vitamin deficiencies, learning a new, effective form of pulsed exercise, or treating chronic viruses with innovative supplements and medicines, most have gotten better. And yet, in spite of all I've learned about the laws of fatigue and the complex weave of its causes, I sometimes wonder why it seems to be the epidemic of our time.

One clue may lie in the derisive name originally given chronic fatigue: "the yuppie flu." Certain sicknesses are so closely linked to the culture of an era that they become metaphors for our darkest fears and anxieties. Consider the plagues that decimated medieval Europe. With their images of corpses and rats in the streets they embodied a perfect vision of medieval hell. Or the famous post-Victorian neurasthenia—a vague epidemic that left its sensitive victims bedridden and weak, suffering from nervous exhaustion. Hardly an important thinker in turn-of-the-century America escaped this disease, from Theodore Roosevelt to William James. In fact, it was supposedly brought on by too much "brain work" and by the pace of "modern" life.

Like neurasthenia in its era, chronic fatigue seems oddly emblematic of our times. A Steve Kelley cartoon in the *San Diego Union* said it all. "It's more than a run-down feeling, Doc," complains the exhausted yuppie on the examining table. "I feel like I've been hit by a BMW." "It's the yuppie flu," the doctor says. "Take a domestic chablis and call me in the morning."

It's funny, of course, but the cartoon says something profound about lifestyle—and expectations. We live in a culture that places unusual, even extraordinary, demands on us. Ten years ago, most stores were not open on Sundays. Now, all over America, Sunday is a day for shopping. There is no longer a notion of the Sabbath, of a day of rest. You can go to the all-night supermarket and get your entire week's food at 3 A.M. And on traditionally sacrosanct holidays like New Year's or Labor Day, stores are open for special clearance sales. Any experience is available to us at any time—whether it's an African safari or an eighty-hour work week—to baby boomers, in particular, who were born in peacetime, into affluence and enormous expectations.

Tired All the Time

Our horizons seem limitless, our choices unbounded. The rhythm of life, which should swing between relaxation and activity, now seems like a perpetual race punctuated by brief intervals of exhausted sleep. A typical review of a new, hot New York City club in the magazine *Vanity Fair* describes the young, handsome co-founder as "a former model who moonlights in real estate before his real job of going out every night."

Those daunting expectations—to work hard, play hard, look good, and enjoy every moment—may be why some of my patients are so desperate. Their fatigue is real and is particularly devastating because they didn't believe that illness would ever touch them. "I did everything right, Dr. Hoffman. I ate well. I exercised; I didn't smoke or drink; I practiced safe sex. Why did this happen to me? Why do I feel so tired? Why, why, why?"

Unlike many doctors, I believe they have a right to ask that question. Ours is an era of tremendous expectations—but also a time of tremendous possibilities. We now know more about the impact of diet on health and illness than ever before. Scientists at major universities are at this moment studying the effect of nutrients on organs and even on cells themselves. We understand better how to assess the risk for disease, and how to prevent it. With the enormous Human Genome Project, which is attempting to map every human gene and thus detect and predict genetic diseases, we may be able to engineer our own health from infancy. Not only will we be able to predict genetically determined diseases, we may also begin to understand tendencies and susceptibilities. Some of us may have inherited unusual needs for certain nutrients, and by bolstering them from childhood we may strengthen our health and avoid the pitfalls of fatigue and illness later in life.

As more sensitive tests measure the function of each system of the body, we develop better means of calibrating those systems. Already we have tremendous information at our fingertips. We know that exercise can strengthen the body and prolong life. We can treat allergies, we can detoxify the body of harmful metals, we have profoundly sensitive tests to determine just where the immune system has gone haywire. Now, more than ever before, we have the weapons and knowledge to get down in the trenches and fight fatigue—and overcome it. Vitality can and should be our inalienable right.

How Did We Get So Tired?

•   •   •

The first—and most important—step you can take to conquer your fatigue is to believe you can. That's why I quoted the Roman sage Seneca at the beginning of this book: It is part of the cure to wish to be cured. Anyone can fight fatigue. There are people with metastatic cancer who embark on marathons. I joke with my patients about amazing granny Mavis Lindgren, an eighty-four-year-old who attracted media attention because she can run most men half her age off their feet. In between Elvis sightings, UFO visitations, and other believe-it-when-you-see-it phenomena, this octogenarian was featured in popular tabloids. She took up marathon running at the tender age of seventy and has competed in fifty-eight marathons since then. Four years ago, when she turned eighty, doctors ran a battery of endurance tests on her that showed she had the health of a college coed. She started walking and jogging at the age of sixty-two, after four bouts of pneumonia prompted her doctors to recommend aerobic exercise.

Mavis Lindgren isn't the only extraordinary example of someone who went from tired to terrific. As you finish the first chapter of this book, give your world-weary body a booster shot of hope. Think of seventy-seven-year-old Dexter Woodford, a retired physicist and cancer survivor, who recently competed in a 28.8-mile swim around the island of Manhattan, through chilly, heavily polluted water. And guess who beat him in the race—finishing seventh? Lucyna Krajewska, a twenty-nine-year-old German who is a double leg amputee.

Remember, no matter how tired you feel today, you are now embarking on your own detective story—to hunt down and eliminate the causes of your fatigue. In this book you will learn how to look for and uncover the hidden clues to your own tiredness. You will be able to put together your own generalized fatigue wheel, where you draw a pie-shaped chart and tackle, one by one, the possible causes of fatigue. As you address each cause (or find out that a particular cause is unrelated to your tiredness), your energy will improve.

Fatigue is rarely due to just a single cause. In this book, you will learn how to assess the quality of your sleep. You will find out if you have hidden allergies, and whether you are sensitive to molds, foods, and chemicals. I will tell you how to test your home for toxins that might be causing fatigue. You'll discover if a lack of sunlight might be contributing to your weariness, whether your diet is suited to your particular metabolism, and how a lack of even one vitamin or mineral can interrupt the energy pathways in your body. You'll learn what makes a muscle cell tired, and how to replenish it. I'll tell you how to find out if you're addicted to stress—and whether you are chemically dependent on your own stress hormones.

You'll learn about your endocrine system, and how to test it to discover if there is a hidden weakness in your thyroid or adrenal glands, or in the hormones regulating your reproductive system. I'll tell you about nutrient therapy to gently recalibrate your hormones. Some of those nutrients include vitamin C, pantothenic acid, licorice extract, ginseng, primrose oil, and fish oil.

You'll learn about a condition called syndrome X, which is now an epidemic, and which may be *the* major risk for heart disease. One of its first symptoms is fatigue. A high-sugar diet can exacerbate it, and take a tremendous toll on your body's metabolic machinery.

Feeling tired every day—or even part of every day—is not inevitable. You don't have to live with it. Like many other medical mysteries, fatigue can yield to a determined and systematic investigation.

2

THE PHYSIOLOGY OF FATIGUE

▼

Fatigued. Worn down. Tired out. Pooped. Bushed. Ragged. Weak.
Spent. Dog-tired. Bone-tired. Dead beat. Done in. Ready to drop.
Weary. Burnt out. More dead than alive.

So what is fatigue anyway? There are lots of words to describe it,
but what is this feeling that seems to permeate your life and rob you
of energy?

QUESTION: What is the purpose of fatigue?

ANSWER: What is the purpose of love?

Translate that as: Nature works in mysterious ways. To provide
us with the impetus to have sex we were given libido, which manifests
itself as the tumult and longing of romantic love. To provide us with
the desire to eat we were given appetite, which manifests itself as
hunger, a painful, gnawing longing for food. And to provide us with
the impetus to rest we were given fatigue, which manifests itself as the
intense longing for sleep.

Fatigue, then, can be good. Without it, you would not know your
limits. You might keep exercising in spite of the fact that your muscles
were producing waste products that need to be released by your body.
You might keep working or partying even though your body needed
sleep in order to replenish and balance itself. In fact, one of the problems of modern life is our constant attempt to drown out the message.
We take aspirin for aches, coffee for weariness, sugar for mid-afternoon
slumps.

In the simplest sense, fatigue is the message your body sends you
when it is stressed—when you need to slow down, relax, recoup. To
understand fatigue, the first notion you need to understand is stress.
Think, for example, of the notion of metal fatigue, a term often used
to describe the stress that slowly wears down bridges. I live in Manhattan, an island ringed by rusting and corroding bridges, many of

which were built in the early twentieth century. Engineers are constantly clambering up the girders and cables of these bridges, measuring the effects of weather, traffic, and time—the cumulative effect of stress called metal fatigue. After calculating the amount of fatigue, they know what to repair.

In the same way, stress on the human body can cause fatigue, even though you may not be aware of the precise connection. Stress proceeds in specific stages—and each stage can have a radically different impact on your body. Although you may be tempted at this moment to skip ahead to chapters on the "hard facts" of fatigue and what you can do about tiredness, this short chapter will lay the groundwork for your understanding of how fatigue works. And that understanding is part of the cure.

Your body is always trying to achieve a state of balance, or what we call homeostasis. Stress—whether from exposure to toxic levels of lead, your boss yelling at you, lack of sleep, or the common cold—disrupts homeostasis.

How does your body respond to that disruption? It was only forty years ago that a medical genius named Hans Selye, of the University of Montreal, hit a bull's-eye that nobody else had even seen. He proposed an elegant and remarkable theory of how the body adjusts to stress—a theory that helps explain everything from the athlete's exhilaration to the cardiac patient's stroke. That theory has revolutionized medical thinking and has been confirmed by thousands of scientific studies. It has also propelled the word *stress* into our popular lexicon.

Quite simply, he proposed that stress can cause the body either to adapt or to break down, depending on the strength of the organism. His theory, called the general adaptation syndrome (GAS), found that the body responds to stress as a stimulus.

It is possible to pass through all the stages of the GAS in a single day—for instance, when a person is severely burned and eventually succumbs to his injuries as the body's defenses collapse. Most often, however, it takes years and even a lifetime to reach the stage of exhaustion, which is a result of exposure to thousands of different stressors. Stress comes in a rainbow of different wrappings. The classic signs of stress have been produced in animals by exposing them to anything from loud noises to blinking lights, heat, cold, electric shock, drugs,

THE STAGES OF STRESS

▼

Stage One: Preadaptation
Before exposure to a stressor, the body is in a quiet, preadapted stage.

Stage Two: Fight or Flight
The stressor acts like an alarm clanging at a fire station. A tiny master gland at the base of the brain, the pituitary, responds to the call to arms. This second stage is known as the *nonadapted alarm stage*.
What happens?

1. The pituitary secretes a hormone called ACTH. This hormone rushes through the blood to the adrenal glands, two small peanut-shaped powerhouses located above the kidneys.
2. The adrenals produce other "stress" hormones, like cortisol and adrenaline, which quickly kick the body into its fight-or-flight stance.
3. The body, primed for emergency action, reacts on all fronts. Proteins are converted into sugar, which is instantly available for energy. Much of it is pumped into the blood—causing the blood-sugar level to soar—and the rest is stored in the liver, like players waiting in the dugout for their turn at bat. At the same time, blood pressure increases, as does the heart rate. Minerals are pulled from the bones, and salt is retained in the body. Large amounts of magnesium, in particular, are excreted in the urine. In a sense, the body "borrows" vital nutrients and minerals from its tissues, in order to meet the demands of stress and maintain homeostasis.

Stage Three: Resistance
As long as the body has no particular susceptibility to the stressor and has adequate raw materials at hand, it can constantly rebuild and repair. This repair stage is known as the *stage of resistance*. Every illness, accident, and trauma causes an intense "alarm" reaction, which disrupts homeostasis, followed by a stage of resistance and repair, when homeostasis is achieved again. During acute stress, your nutritional requirements may skyrocket. If your needs are met, and you can satisfy the intense demands of your body's fight-or-flight mobilization, little harm is done.

(continued)

Stage Four: Adaptation

That sounds straightforward enough. What happens, however, if the body is exposed to the same stress again and again? It tries to adapt to the stressor so that the alarm doesn't continually disrupt it. The body automatically resets itself to a new, higher setpoint of alarm. It can't "hear" the stressor anymore. The result? It can maintain homeostasis and freedom from symptoms, despite the ongoing presence of the stressor.

This *adapted stage* will initially not harm a healthy individual—in other words, as long as there is no significant, permanent tissue damage or nutritional depletion, the person will feel healthy. In fact, the body may actually become habituated to the presence of the stressor—and come to "need" it to maintain homeostasis. This can account for the well-known phenomenon called "masked addiction," in which a person craves the very substance that is actually stressing the body. A good example is the craving many people experience for coffee—when in fact the caffeine is sapping the adrenals as well as important chemicals in the brain, and can actually be the cause of periodic headaches, heartburn, and fatigue.

Stage Five: Maladaptation

Unfortunately, the adaptation process can go awry. Adaptation is harmful when the body's stores are depleted. When stress is constant and prolonged, extraordinary demands are made, especially, on the liver, cardiovascular system, and adrenals. Critical minerals like magnesium may become chronically depleted. The nervous system and the immune system suffer. A person enters the next stage, called *maladaptation*.

In maladaptation, an individual begins to show signs and symptoms of stress. *One of the cardinal symptoms is fatigue.* This is because some biologic pathway is overwhelmed or damaged. It may be as simple as not having enough of a single nutrient that is needed to produce stress hormones. For instance, the need for vitamin C soars during stress. With serious vitamin-C deficiency—true scurvy—the adrenal glands actually undergo tiny hemorrhages, and their production of hormones is significantly lowered. The symptoms of classic scurvy are bleeding gums, exhaustion, and lassitude.

Stage Six: Switching

The signs of maladaptation can be enormously varied—and can show up in any organ. Sometimes, in fact, the body will seem to target one

(continued)

The Physiology of Fatigue

organ for a while (a person may suffer asthma attacks) and then spare that organ and seem to target another (the person may then suffer from chronic irritable bowel). This is called *switching*. Maladaptation symptoms can range from chronic tiredness to a rash to inflammation in every joint of the body. Though most of us think of symptoms as the sign of illness caused by a specific virus or bacteria, they are usually the sign of the body's reaction to stress. That reaction is experienced as disease. Even so, this "disease" process shows that the body is still actively attempting to repair itself—inflammation, fever, and discomfort are actually the signs of the body's resistance to a stressor that is overwhelming it.

Stage Seven: Exhaustion
If maladaptation persists, and is acute enough, the last and most tragic stage of adaptation occurs. It is known as *the stage of exhaustion*. At this point, one or more systems in the body have completely lost their ability to recover from a particular stress. The individual experiences constant, chronic symptoms that are unrelated to the stressor and result from nutrient exhaustion or irreversible damage to tissues. Repair mechanisms have completely failed.

chemicals, viruses, bacteria, surgery, burns, fasting, toxins, or suboptimal diets—even by forced, prolonged exercise.

How does the general adaptation syndrome work in real life? Consider the cigarette smoker. For most people, the initial experience of a cigarette is devastating. It is painful to draw harsh, toxic smoke into your lungs, and the body responds to the alarm with violent coughing. The stomach recoils with nausea and blood vessels constrict, producing headaches. However, after repeated exposures, you adapt and even find smoking pleasurable. You become habituated to the nicotine and come to crave it. In fact, you soon perceive smoking as a necessary pleasure, and the lack of a cigarette as a stressor. Cigarette smoking becomes addictive, and the smoker is caught in a cycle of alternating irritability and satisfaction. For a long time, the body seems "adapted" and symptoms seem minimal. Eventually, however, they begin to appear. The happy smoker becomes the smoker with headaches, poorly defined malaise, a constant cough, wheezing, mood swings, and frequent sinus infections. Eventually, he may have irreparable organ damage (such as emphysema), and once he reaches a state of exhaustion, he may develop lung cancer and die.

Another, more insidious example of GAS? Take a child who is allergic to wheat but whose allergy is "masked" because she eats wheat products every day. She may experience occasional headaches or sleepiness, but her mother doesn't connect them to wheat. If she does not have wheat for several weeks, her body will go through withdrawal and deadaptation, and return to the setpoint of homeostasis it experienced before she ever ate wheat. Then she eats a big plate of whole-wheat pasta. Within half an hour she becomes agitated and hyperactive. Her body is in the alarm stage. Later in the day she gets a splitting headache—maladaptation. She sleeps fitfully, but when she wakes the next day, feels fine: her body has repaired its systems, and she is once more in homeostasis.

Now that you understand a little about the nature of stress, let's take a trip down the energy cascade in the body. How is energy produced, and where does it go?

Walt Whitman may have said it best: "I sing the body electric," he proclaimed. The biggest energy consumer in the body is the cell, and it functions much as an electric battery does. The one thing that distinguishes life from death in that cell is its ability to keep certain chemicals outside and other chemicals inside. The cell is a biological battery, using the electrical charge of these nutrients to give it the energy it needs to live. It must continually push back waves of sodium and calcium and try to retain its stores of potassium and magnesium. In this way, the cell manages to keep a positive charge inside and a negative charge outside, much like a battery. People think of cells as little fluid-filled plastic bags, but in fact they are more like living organisms enclosed in a force field. That force field requires a huge amount of energy to pump nutrients into and out of the cell.

The cells that need the most energy are those of the brain. The brain's metabolism is about 7.5 times the average metabolism for the rest of the body. You may be surprised to learn that brain cells use far more energy than the heart, which pumps blood throughout the entire body.

The Physiology of Fatigue

The main source of energy for the body's dance of life is sugar. Plants, by the way, convert the sun's energy into sugar through a very complex cycle, and they use the nutrients in the soil to help. For humans, sugar comes in many forms in food (as fructose in fruit, as complex chains of sugars in whole grains, as sucrose in table sugar), and in the body, it is broken down into glucose. Breaking down sugars releases energy. The cell is so efficient at this process that the body as a whole is able to utilize 66 percent of the energy available to it. Compare that with the finest racing car, which at best utilizes about 20 percent of its fuel.

Through a chain of steps called the Krebs cycle, that energy is locked onto a chemical called ATP. The Krebs cycle is the nemesis of every freshman medical student—a complex chain of thirty-two reactions that students are often forced to memorize. It was discovered by a German researcher named Ernest Krebs, who won the Nobel Prize for describing this essential series of energy reactions in the body. ATP stands for adenosine triphosphate, and it is basically a series of high-energy phosphorus atoms that are bound to a carrier molecule. ATP is the intracellular currency of energy. When ATP is broken down, the freed bonds release energy.

Think of the body as a dam system harnessing a mighty river. The river is a metaphor for the burning of sugar, which can occur with fierce and uncontrolled intensity. There is obviously tremendous energy in that river, and as it rushes through the body it is channeled into little hydroelectric stations that transform it or store it. At each power station are little chemical messengers waiting to shuttle off the valuable ATP that has been generated. It is as if the chaos had been broken down and harnessed into tiny cellular explosions of energy. That energy can be stored as fat or put into usable morsels. Vitamins and minerals are catalysts in these energy reactions.

One of the most important "energy stations" in the cell is the mitochondrion. It's the power pack, or tiny electric generator, in the cell. Mitochondria convert fuel into energy and depend in particular on two substances: coenzyme Q-10 (also known as ubiquinone, because it is ubiquitous in the body), which helps transport electrons through the energy cascade, and carnitine, an amino acid that helps shuttle fat into the mitochondrion. Mitochondria are especially dense in muscle cells, and when you look at the muscles of elite athletes under a microscope, they have many more mitochondria than those of an average person.

Every part of your body needs ATP. It is the basic building block of all energy reactions. In addition, there are certain substances, aside from carnitine and ubiquinone, that are absolutely crucial to the energy pathway. For instance, most of the B vitamins are intimately involved in the transfer of energy.

You may wonder why, if ATP is the source of energy, you can't simply take it in a pill. Unfortunately, if you try to take ATP as a supplement it is broken down by your digestive system before it can ever reach the cell, where it is needed. However, one interesting experiment has used ATP bound to magnesium in an intravenous drip in cases of cardiogenic shock, a state of profound energy shutdown where all cellular processes become slowed prior to death. In animals with cardiogenic shock, intravenous magnesium ATP prolonged life.

The physiology of fatigue is a subject as vast as a continent, but here are some of the questions my patients most often ask me, with my answers:

Why does the body need oxygen for energy?

Just like a fire, your body uses oxygen to burn your fuel, which is sugar. Oxygenation of tissue is crucial; that's why people with circulation problems also have energy problems: not enough oxygen is being carried into the tissue.

Think of one of the most common causes of oxygen deprivation, carbon-monoxide poisoning. The telltale symptom is fatigue, along with confusion and malaise, and finally stupor and death. Émile Zola was said to have died while writing because of carbon monoxide poisoning from a malfunctioning stove. What happens? Carbon monoxide fills up the receptors for oxygen on your hemoglobin, the oxygen-carrying substance within your red blood cells. Little oxygen is transported to your starved tissues. What is fascinating is that cigarette smoke—even downstream "passive" smoke from a nearby cigarette—contains substantial amounts of carbon monoxide. Whenever I hear a smoker tell me he is fatigued, I insist that he quit the habit before I evaluate his complaint of tiredness.

Why does low blood sugar make me feel tired?

The Physiology of Fatigue

Sugar is the source of fuel in the body. It is stored in the form of fat, or a form of sugar called glycogen, which is in the muscles and the liver. Glycogen can be used up in a few hours. When athletes train, their muscles gain a greater capacity to store glycogen. That is why you have to build up your capacity for an endurance event like a marathon.

The brain, above all, requires sugar as fuel. However, after periods of starvation it can be made to burn ketones, which are by-products of fat metabolism. This may have been a lifesaving adaptation for primitive man during times of famine, because the brain could survive on ketones released from body fat. That's one reason fasting may be difficult at first, until ketone metabolism kicks in. Because blood sugar is steady during ketone metabolism, you can feel a certain easy euphoria, although you may not have much strength. I've run while fasting, but it's like a little, gentle lope. There is no power or endurance, but there is a real mental clarity because you are not buffeted by the urgent needs of changing blood-sugar levels.

Is fatigue in the body or the mind?

This is a central question for fatigue-ologists, and it could be reframed this way: Is fatigue central or peripheral? Does it start in tired muscles or in a "tired" brain?

The answer is both. A long-term study at the University of Connecticut School of Medicine's Fatigue Clinic found that depression was the cause of chronic fatigue in over half of 277 participants. Conversely, a day's hard physical labor can leave your muscles tired and your brain fatigued.

Even so, the interweaving of mind and body is far more complex. For instance, there can be profound mental adaptation to regular exercise. When I ran my first marathon I was almost ready to give up after three miles. I already had countless aches and pains. The mere thought of the overwhelming distance ahead of me was fatiguing. But by about mile ten, I had a sense of incredible euphoria as my body's own endorphins kicked in. I felt borne along on the tide of my body's own feel-good chemicals. When I hit mile twenty-four, I had completely run out of fuel, and it was only sheer willpower—mind over matter—that pushed me those last two miles. A few minutes after I had finished, I was exhilarated again, awash in endorphins.

Why do I get tired in mid-afternoon?

Tired All the Time

There can be many reasons, including a dip in blood sugar, or postmeal drowsiness. Humans also have natural biological rhythms that program when they tend to be sleepy or to feel awake. Most of us are programmed to drowse in the mid-afternoon, and the famous siesta was probably invented to cope with this phenomenon.

Why do my muscles feel tired and achy after I exercise?

As the muscles pump, stretch, and contract during exercise, they burn a lot of fuel to make energy. The toxic by-product of that fuel is known as lactic acid, and your body has to cart it away, detoxify it in the liver, and then reutilize it. If you are exercising strenuously, some of the lactic acid builds up in your muscles, causing achiness and fatigue.

Lactic acid is actually the by-product of muscles that are working in the absence of oxygen. They are functioning in an anaerobic, or oxygen-starved, environment. That's when you get the "burn." You've gone beyond your threshold, and your body is functioning without an adequate oxygen supply. In a brisk walk, by comparison, you don't force yourself beyond that threshold.

Why does aerobic exercise ultimately increase energy?

First, it increases circulation, so the blood can bring more oxygen to all parts of the body. Second, it speeds up the metabolism, so you are functioning at a higher setpoint. Third, exercise actually increases the number of mitochondria, the energy powerhouses, in the body. After exercising for a few months, you have significantly more mitochondria. Your aerobic threshold is higher, and you are able to use oxygen to liberate energy. In the absence of oxygen, an energy process occurs that is far less efficient. It is similar to a primitive process in certain yeasts and bacteria called anaerobic glycolysis—the breakdown of sugar in the absence of oxygen. The price is lactic acid production and consequent fatigue.

How does the body signal that it is tired?

The body and the brain use chemical messengers known as neurotransmitters. Some of these signal the body to slow down, and they are called inhibitory neurotransmitters. Others signal body processes to speed up. These chemical messengers are called excitatory neurotransmitters.

Why can't medical science invent a neurotransmitter that gives me energy?

The Physiology of Fatigue

Because the body is not that simple. The neural sequences are vastly complicated and one sequence may be dependent on ten or twenty others. For instance, some inhibitory neurotransmitters actually inhibit the slowdown process and so indirectly cause excitation.

Even so, providing the body and brain with more of a certain neurotransmitter is the basis of psychopharmacology. By giving patients certain drugs that change levels of brain neurotransmitters or supply them with neurotransmitters they may lack, we are trying to give them energy and a sense of well-being. The difficulty with that approach is clear in patient response: you may have to try many different drugs to improve mood, and you may get only a partial, imperfect response. In addition, the drug may stop working after a while. We don't have the magic bullet. Prozac, a popular antidepressant, was initially hailed as just such a panacea. It helped many patients, didn't work for others, and seemed to cause severe depression and pronounced side effects in some patients.

Why is it that if I think about being tired, I feel more tired?

A lot of our experience of life depends on our interpretation of events. If you identify a bodily sensation as a headache, it isn't so bad. If you imagine it's a fatal brain tumor, it may start hurting a lot! Similarly, if you are constantly monitoring and interpreting your internal state, and worrying about fatigue, you may "feel" more tired than you are. Studies show that certain of us are hard-wired to be more attuned to our sensations. Those people are called "amplifiers." Not only do they feel internal sensations of pain and pleasure more intensely, they are more attuned to differences in external stimuli, like colors.

Why do I get tired after I eat?

The involuntary nervous system has two "parts" or divisions. One is called sympathetic. In sympathetic arousal we're geared for fight or flight, so digestion becomes a superfluous activity. People feel highly energized but digestion slows. That's why people who are extremely nervous don't want to eat, or if they do eat, they feel as if food were stuck in their craw and they experience gastric upset. In a parasympathetic state, digestion is better, and peristalsis occurs more readily. Blood is shunted toward the digestive organs and away from the heart and brain. Digestion shifts your body to a parasympathetic state, and so you may feel somewhat lethargic.

In addition, when you eat a meal high in carbohydrates, you tend to increase brain levels of a neurotransmitter called serotonin. Serotonin is known to make people feel calm, even sleepy.

Why do allergies make me feel fatigued?

Nobody is exactly sure, but we do know that histamine is released in an allergic reaction. Histamine causes inflammation (such as a welt, hive, swollen nasal passages). Researchers have recently discovered that histamine also functions as a brain neurotransmitter. Perhaps it is part of a chemical cascade that causes you to slow down and rest.

We aren't yet sure of all the functions of histamine in the brain, but it's so powerful that recently a patent has been obtained for the use of a potent antihistamine used in stomach ulcers. Called Zantac, it is being considered as a drug to help block histamine in the brains of schizophrenic patients. This use was virtually foreseen by the work of a controversial physician named Karl Pfeiffer, the late head of the Princeton Bio-Brain Center. He estimated that a considerable percentage of schizophrenics had hidden food allergies, called "cerebral" allergies. According to Pfeiffer, histamine was a crucial mediator in the illness.

Why do I get tired when I'm sick?

Part of the reason may be that the immune system releases chemicals that can cause fatigue. One interesting study suggested this. Patients receiving special immunotherapy for cancer found themselves feeling unusually fatigued and depressed—so much so that a psychiatrist was required to be part of the study team. These patients were given a type of natural substance called lymphokines, which activate the body's white blood cells. While receiving their immune boost, the patients also felt lethargic and sad. This may seem bewildering, but perhaps part of the body's wisdom is to create an immune system that when triggered into action by an invading virus or bacteria, also creates fatigue. The fatigue causes the person to rest, and that means the body can conserve its energy to fight the invader.

Are some people born energetic, and others born tired?

Some people seem to need a lot of sleep, and others can flourish on a few hours' sleep a night. Genetics plays a powerful role in your levels of energy and how much sleep you require. We can see this in the habits of different species: sloths and opossums spend eighteen to twenty hours every day sleeping in trees. Deer and antelope sleep two to three hours at a time. Hummingbirds are known to have great bursts of activity, burning fuel at an incredible rate and quickly becoming completely exhausted. Think of yourself, your family and friends. Aren't some of us hummingbirds, others antelopes, and still others opossums?

It's possible that some people are parasympathetic-dominant, while others are sympathetic-dominant. This means that one part of their nervous system dominates (just as some people are right-handed and others favor their left hand). People who are parasympathetic-dominant tend to be laid back and less energetic. People who are governed by their sympathetic nervous system may be cerebral live wires who can sustain high levels of physical activity and mental concentration.

Can vitamins and minerals make you more energetic?

They can certainly play an important role in boosting energy, especially where there are deficiencies in critical nutrients in the energy pathway. Remember that stress is the beginning of fatigue—stress depletes us of nutrients and minerals.

Vitamins, minerals, and enzymes are known as assistants, or co-factors, in energy reactions. When your body is poisoned, whether by radiation, pesticides, pollution, toxic metals, viruses, bacteria, or any other toxins, these vitamin, enzyme, and mineral helpers are often "uncoupled," or broken away from the energy cascade. A reaction somewhere along the chain doesn't occur normally, and it can derail the entire process. When your system is loaded with these toxic un-couplers, energy production slows down, causing profound fatigue.

A remarkable example of how this uncoupling can be reversed is seen in chelation therapy (see Chapter 8), a process that pulls toxic metals from the body. These metals, stored in cells and circulating in the blood, may have uncoupled many steps along the energy cascade. Once they have been removed, people often feel a burst of energy. They go from tired, foggy, fuzzy, and achy to feeling newly energized.

It seems like I've been tired for years. What could be the reason?

Read this book!

3

THE INTRICATE INTERPLAY OF HORMONES

▼

One of the most common unrecognized causes of fatigue is hormonal imbalance. Your delicate hormonal system can easily be disrupted—by stress, lifestyle, drugs, or nutritional deficiencies. And a common sign of hormonal disruption is—you guessed it—unremitting fatigue. I see it commonly in my practice, and I often find that it has gone undiagnosed by other doctors.

I sometimes wish I had become an endocrinologist. This special kind of doctor is above all a detective, a thinker and a sleuth who performs subtle tests and offers equally "subtle" treatment—and yet the results can be almost miraculous. If ever I were to wake up one nightmare morning and find that my own field of nutritional medicine had shut down, like some vast department-store chain that overnight went out of business, I'd opt to be an endocrinologist. More aggressive and decisive physicians—such as the cardiothoracic surgeon, with his dramatic, lifesaving interventions—probably consider the endocrinologist a ponderous analytical slowpoke. A gastroenterologist has a whole arsenal of instruments with which he can scope every inch of your GI tract. A cardiologist can dazzle his patients with high-tech tools to invade and examine the arterial walls themselves. There's nothing much the endocrinologist can do except take a lab test. Endocrinology, by contrast with the more "dramatic" specialties, is a quiet labor of love.

And yet, it is absolutely essential. The endocrine system is the ultimate regulator of your well-being, and treating endocrine problems can be one of the most satisfying activities in medicine. Take a patient who is mysteriously ill, and who is told that she is depressed and in all likelihood imagining the vast array of symptoms from which she suffers. Often an endocrinologist does something as simple as draw a tube of blood, and based on careful interpretation of the results, administers a minute amount of a medication that is a copy of a chemical already in the body. That is the ultimate in gentle medicine, and the patient can find her life transformed. It's downright elegant.

The actual technology is amazingly sophisticated. Endocrinology took a giant leap forward in the 1970s, when Rosalyn Yalow and her husband perfected an astonishingly sensitive way of measuring the very minute amounts of hormones that circulate in the body. This technique, called radioimmunoassay (RIA) revolutionized the field and won Dr. Yalow a Nobel Prize. Now we can measure when a hormone's level is off kilter by a few millionths of a gram, and we have proof that such impossibly subtle changes can cause disruptive symptoms in every organ of the body, from dry skin to heart palpitations and muscle degeneration.

Hormones, indeed, are the master regulators of well-being. In this chapter, I'll take a look at one very common hormonal cause of exhaustion: thyroid malfunction. In a practice where I feature the care of chronic fatigue, thyroid problems show up in about 10 percent of my patients, and treating hidden thyroid problems can be both tricky and hugely rewarding. Both excess *and* insufficient thyroid hormone can cause profound fatigue. I'll explain just how often doctors may miss thyroid malfunction, how to perform self-tests at home, and then which tests to ask your doctor for. I'll tell you which therapies are safe and how certain herbs and lifestyle changes can boost stressed glands.

Before you can begin to assess the health of your own hormones, you should understand just what a hormone means to the body. It is the chemical secretion of a gland. There are two types of glands: endocrine and exocrine. The latter produce nonhormone substances that are secreted into the digestive tract, like pancreatic enzymes, or are exuded through pores in the skin, like sweat. By contrast, each endocrine gland fires its own hormones straight into the bloodstream, and these hormones rush through the body, sending messages that speed up or slow down body processes. How does a gland know when to release a hormone? Our hormones are linked in a delicate and complex web of interactions—they are stimulated by certain chemical messengers and inhibited by others. Hormones help regulate our whole internal world, from how fast we burn up calories in food, to how quickly we grow, how well we repair wounds, and, of course, when we reach puberty.

Without a healthy balance of hormones, a person can literally feel so fatigued life doesn't seem worth living. That happened to a patient of mine who had the most severe hormone deficiency I have ever encountered. I still remember how Shelley sat slumped in a chair on her first visit, her face lined with unhappiness, and recited in a dull monotone, "I used to teach dance full time, Dr. Hoffman." Now she raised her head and said with effort, "I feel incredibly fatigued, and I'm so depressed, and all the doctors can tell me is I'm going through premature menopause and I have to live with it."

She was forty-four years old; three years earlier she had begun experiencing sporadic menstrual periods. Since then, she had been suffering from devastating fatigue, body aches, and malaise. She had gained a great deal of weight and felt totally depleted. Seven different specialists hadn't helped; the last had put her on estrogen-replacement therapy and recommended a psychotherapist.

The estrogen didn't help much. And even the best therapy, Shelley protested, wasn't going to help her "adjust" to this terrible chronic exhaustion.

Shelley turned out to be one of my most fascinating, mysterious, and ultimately successful cases. When I first examined her that day, thyroid malfunction popped into my mind. But I was disappointed when her thyroid tests came back. Usually when you suffer from low thyroid, you have elevated levels of thyroid-stimulating hormone (TSH)—a product of the pituitary gland—in the blood. That's because the pituitary is desperately signaling the thyroid to pump out more thyroxin, the thyroid's "energy" hormone. Shelley, however, had low TSH levels.

Perhaps, I reasoned, her adrenals were underactive. I wondered if she might be suffering from Addison's disease, the classic wasting-away syndrome that occurs when the adrenal glands stop functioning.

"Shelley," I said, "I'm going to ask you to see a top endocrinologist I know." A week later the endocrinologist called me. He was incredibly excited. "Ron, this is one of the most curious cases you'll ever see! This woman is suffering from a failure of all her hormones. The cause is a benign tumor in her pituitary gland, which has completely disrupted the activity of the gland." Noting a peculiar pattern in her tests, he had ordered an MRI scan of her brain, and he discovered a small benign tumor that didn't require surgery but needed to be watched.

The pituitary gland is the master regulator, the control station for the whole endocrine system. It orchestrates the activity of all other glands in the body. Because Shelley's pituitary had stopped functioning, three whole systems in her body had failed: her thyroid, her adrenal glands, and her ovaries. The pituitary's failure explained her puzzling test results: for instance, there was no extra TSH in her blood because the pituitary wasn't releasing it, as usually happens in low-thyroid conditions.

No wonder Shelley felt like the walking dead. She was bankrupt of all hormones. We put her on a regimen of five replacement hormones: estrogen, progesterone, thyroid, and two adrenal hormones. And almost immediately she began to improve.

Shelley is an incredible example of the power of hormones: Without them, she felt as exhausted and lifeless as a rag doll. Two years later she is feeling vibrant and energetic and has resumed her old teaching schedule.

Along with the many diseases of modern man, such as heart disease and cancer, count thyroid malfunction. Thyroid disease—both hyperactive and underactive—is so extraordinarily prevalent today that even by conservative estimates it may strike up to 15 percent of the adult population. Women are particularly susceptible, and the disease seems to run in families, but even so we don't know why it is on the rise. One reason may be that the thyroid doesn't have built-in surplus capacity, like the liver or kidneys. Even when 90 percent of the liver is removed in surgery, the 10 percent remaining can suffice—and it can regenerate. But if thyroid capacity declines, through the wear and tear of life itself, the symptoms can be profound.

The thyroid, along with the adrenals, is probably the gland most susceptible to the tremendous stress of a fast-paced existence. According to one study of 219 patients suffering from newly diagnosed Graves' disease (a form of hyperthyroidism), negative and stressful life events were strongly linked to thyroid disease. A typical thyroid patient? George Bush, under fantastic pressure during the Gulf War, who was

The Intricate Interplay of Hormones

going, going, going, to the point where his thyroid began to race like a hot rod gunned by a teenage boy—pouring out excess hormone until he suffered atrial fibrillation (a frightening, chaotic flutter of the heart muscle) while jogging. (His wife, Barbara, also suffers from this disease, and their dog, Millie, has suffered health problems. Some doctors speculate there may be a single environmental cause of the family illness.)

Another possible reason for the increase in thyroid disease is the high prevalence of autoimmune disease today. Immunity in general is being assaulted by toxic chemicals in food, water, and air. Several forms of thyroid imbalance are the result of "autoimmune" problems, where the thyroid becomes inflamed, produces too much hormone, and then in exhaustion finally sputters out.

When the thyroid malfunctions, it may produce excess thyroid hormone (hyperthyroid), or it may degenerate and produce too little (hypothyroid). Answer the following questions to determine if you might be hyperthyroid:

Could You Be Hyperthyroid?

1. Do you feel wired but tired? Are you exhausted and yet jittery, as if you've perpetually drunk too much coffee?
2. Have you lost weight recently for no apparent reason?
3. Do you have trouble sleeping?
4. Do you suffer from heart palpitations?
5. Does your resting pulse race?
6. Do your hands shake? Extend your arms and hold a piece of paper. The fine tremor of a hyperthyroid's hand will be magnified.
7. Do your eyes bulge? This is symptomatic of one type of hyperthyroid condition, Graves' disease.
8. Do you feel heat-intolerant and sweat a lot?

Could You Be Hypothyroid?

In contrast, the hypothyroid patient produces too little thyroid hormone, and the symptoms are much different. Ask yourself the following questions:

1. Are you depressed, lethargic, and easily chilled? Are you the person who is always asking someone to close the window because you're cold?

2. Do you gain weight easily?

3. Do you suffer from chronic fatigue?

4. Do you have dry skin, hair loss, eczema, or adult acne?

5. Do you suffer from muscle aches, constipation, and hoarseness?

6. Do you have PMS or menstrual abnormalities? Is your libido low?

7. Are your feet and legs swollen and your nails brittle?

8. Do you get a lot of colds and flu? One cardinal "unseen" symptom of low thyroid is increased vulnerability to infection.

As common as thyroid disease may be, it often goes unnoticed by many doctors and patients. Thyroid specialist Stephen Langer, M.D., author of *Solved: The Riddle of Illness* (Keats Publishers), counts over one hundred known symptoms of thyroid deficiency. It has even been linked to susceptibility to cancer.

I am always surprised by the misconceptions my patients bring into the office. They aren't sure what the thyroid gland does except speed up the heart and help people lose weight. In the most basic sense, every cell in the body is affected by the thyroid, since thyroid hormone regulates the rate at which energy is consumed by the cells. Before you go on, pause to look over these common myths about the thyroid in the box on pages 43 and 44.

Many people with a "normal" thyroid test have what is known as "subclinical" hypothyroidism, and so they walk away from their doctor's offices believing their thyroid is normal.

One famous crusader against hidden thyroid problems is Broda Barnes, who views low thyroid as the number-one cause of chronic fatigue. Barnes discovered that most of his tired patients had unusually low early-morning body temperatures, often below 97.8 degrees. Low temperature is common in hypothyroidism (as well as a few other conditions, such as low adrenal function). When Dr. Barnes treated his patients with thyroid, he was astonished at the remarkable improvement many of them experienced. Barnes was criticized by conventional endocrinologists because he did not conduct a double-blind experiment, and so had no control for the placebo effect (which can

FACTS AND FALLACIES OF THYROID FUNCTION

▼

Myth: Iodine is good for the thyroid, so if you want to protect your thyroid, or even to increase thyroid activity, just take lots of kelp, which is rich in iodine.

Fact: Iodine is essential for thyroid function, but the type of hypothyroidism that results from lack of iodine is extraordinarily rare in the Western world. It was prevalent at a time when isolated rural areas of the country had no produce that was grown in coastal, iodine-rich soils. Today, diners in Albuquerque can enjoy grilled tuna flown in that morning from the ocean, and people in Duluth can eat jumbo Gulf shrimp. Moreover, many foods are liberally flavored with iodized salts, and many restaurants and fast-food eateries rely on iodine solutions to sanitize their kitchen equipment. Iodine consumption these days in this country is often high. Excess iodine may even depress thyroid function, as has been shown in certain Japanese who consume large amounts of iodine-rich seaweed.

Myth: Thyroid medication is good for helping you lose weight and for combating depression.

Fact: These problems are unacceptable indications for dispensing thyroid medication—even though, until the last decade, well-meaning physicians often gave thyroid hormone to patients as a panacea. One has only to see a patient who is hyperthyroid to realize that the mere addition of thyroid doesn't make you feel good. Despite racing thyroids, these patients are often exhausted all the time, like amphetamine or caffeine addicts. Worse yet, a recent study showed that unnecessary excess thyroid supplementation may accelerate the loss of bone, known as osteoporosis.

Myth: Overweight people who seem to eat little invariably have low thyroids to blame.

Fact: Though low thyroid is one cause of obesity in people who can't lose weight, even on a diet, the most common cause is a hereditary tendency to obesity, coupled with yo-yo dieting. Crash dieting slows the body's metabolic rate to a crawl. And as soon as one goes off a stringent diet, weight gain is likely. This is because of the body's exquisitely programmed adaptation to feast and famine. It worked well for the paleolithic hunter-gatherer, but today we are "stone-agers in

(continued)

the fast lane," to borrow a phrase from Melvin Konner, a co-author of *The Paleolithic Prescription.*

Myth: Hypothyroidism is basically a woman's disease.

Fact: Though women suffer from low thyroid function far more often than men, the ratio is 4 to 1. Women are more susceptible to autoimmune diseases, including thyroid problems. It may be that men are protected by higher levels of androgens, the male hormones, in their blood. Nonetheless, hypothyroidism remains a significant over-looked cause of fatigue in men.

Myth: Cold hands are a giveaway sign of hypothyroidism.

Fact: Cold hands may be a symptom of this disorder, but most often they are a sign of an imbalance in the autonomic nervous system. The sympathetic nervous system—which is responsible for the fight-or-flight syndrome—often overreacts in certain people under stress, causing cold hands and feet.

Myth: Taking thyroid hormone will "fix" your thyroid.

Fact: Though some people regard thyroid medication as a tem-porary panacea that will help them get rid of a problem condition, taking thyroid hormone is usually a lifetime proposition. It replaces thyroid that your own gland simply doesn't make. The occasional ex-ception is an overweight person who is borderline low thyroid and takes thyroid hormone. Feeling energized, this person may then diet and exercise, and lose weight. When the thyroid has less body mass to fuel, its borderline levels may suffice, and the person can stop taking supplemental thyroid medication.

be as high as 33 percent). Even so, his approach has revolutionized the attitudes of many physicians.

Dr. Barnes's basal body temperature test is a simple, at-home test that provides a valuable clue to thyroid disease. You simply shake down a thermometer before going to bed at night and leave it on the bedside table. Any type of thermometer will do. As soon as you awake in the morning, insert the thermometer snugly in your armpit for ten minutes as you lie quietly in bed. Do not get up until you are done taking this measurement. Record your results for three consecutive mornings. Results averaging less than 97.4 suggest hypothyroidism.

Women obtain the most accurate readings when they are not menstruating.

Another valuable and old-fashioned test is the Achilles'-heel reflex test, which I measure by a "photomotogram," also known as a Kinemometer. It's an old-fashioned device once relied on by endocrinologists to measure precisely the slowing of reflexes that occurs with hypothyroidism. The heel is tapped, and the machine records a graph image of the reflex response. A slowed response is not always indicative of thyroid disease (for instance, peripheral nerve damage caused by alcoholism can give the same response), but it is a valuable clue. I find these two tests particularly useful once I've started prescribing thyroid hormone. It gives me a measure of the most important thing: patient response to the hormone.

Suppose you've looked at the symptoms of thyroid malfunction and you think you may be suffering from them. What do you do next? What do you tell your doctor? What tests do you ask for? What if he says your tests are normal and shows you the door?

First, understand that if it is not easy to talk to your doctor, it may not be your fault. A recent study of more than a thousand encounters between internists and their patients at a health-maintenance organization found that most people are interrupted by their doctors within the first eighteen seconds of describing what is bothering them. And often the patient, feeling a little unsure or shy, leaves his most important complaint for last. According to Richard Frankel, who helped conduct the study, "The physician has his or her hand on the doorknob, saying, 'Do you have any more questions?' and shaking the patient's hand. . . . The patient will say, 'Yeah, as a matter of fact, I've been feeling blue and life isn't worth living.' " Doctors tend to regard this eleventh-hour "confession" as a hidden agenda on the part of a manipulative patient. The truth may be that the doctor interrupted the patient earlier in the encounter, or perhaps didn't allow for the difficulties some patients have articulating what's *really* bothering them.

On the other hand, patients who approach the doctor with a list of symptoms and questions may not get the response they want either. Studies show that lists are irritating to many doctors; they tend to regard such patients as hypochondriacs. I myself welcome a list because I think it bespeaks an organized patient, but I'm not typical. In fact, doctors refer disparagingly to list makers as patients who suffer from *la maladie du petit papier* (the sickness of the little piece of paper). Therefore, if you feel you need a list, let your doctor know that it will allow you to speak more clearly and quickly about your condition.

One good approach is to think about the questions you want answered and have five or six of them prepared in your mind before you go to the office. Bring a notepad to take notes.

This may sound like simplistic advice, but a study of hundreds of patients at the New England Medical Center in Boston found that diabetic and hypertensive patients who were coached on taking more control during their doctors' visits had a *measurable* drop in their blood-sugar levels and blood pressure six months later.

Once you have voiced your concerns to your doctor, be prepared for him to give you a warning about thyroid medicine: that it is not a panacea for fatigue. Don't be surprised. Few doctors are fatigue-ologists. Most prefer not to deal with as perplexing and subtle a symptom as fatigue. If you haven't been checked for thyroid thoroughly and the symptoms I've suggested seem to point in the direction of a thyroid malfunction, just suggest politely but persistently that additional tests be ordered. (Unfortunately, some doctors feel their authority has been usurped by such a suggestion, and they may refuse to order these tests. Doctors like to feel like independent investigators. Usually, nonetheless, they will agree to further testing if there is a reasonable possibility of a disorder.)

I hope that in the future more sensitive thyroid tests will be developed. Just as tests for sugar metabolism and insulin resistance have become finely tuned (see Chapter 5), we need more sensitive tests to assess the possibility of thyroid malfunction. One uncommon test that I am fond of is the TRH (thyroid-releasing hormone) stimulation test. It's almost like a stress test for the thyroid, for it measures the pituitary gland's response to a hormone secreted by the hypothalamus. The dynamic interaction of pituitary, hypothalamus, and thyroid can then be studied. Ask your doctor about it.

Another intriguing and useful test detects the presence of antibodies the body has manufactured against the thyroid gland itself. These autoantibodies tell you when you're headed for thyroid trouble, since they indicate an inflammatory condition of the thyroid. Sometimes patients with normal blood levels of thyroid hormone have significant levels of autoantibodies, which may indicate that the thyroid is under attack and is fighting to maintain adequate levels. Giving a little thyroid hormone can help the thyroid rest, and adding anti-inflammatory nutrients such as essential fatty acids and vitamins may help soothe the inflamed gland.

Suppose your doctor agrees: You have a thyroid problem. Your gland isn't functioning effectively, or perhaps your body isn't absorbing the hormone properly. You need medication. What should you take? How much? Will you need to take it for life?

Prescribing thyroid is an art. Each person responds differently, and tests often rely on the presence of thyroid hormone circulating in the blood. That is a little like deciding whether diabetics need insulin by measuring their insulin levels. Instead, we measure blood-sugar levels. In fact, the treatment of diabetes offers a profoundly important clue to the treatment of thyroid disease. One of the key concepts in diabetes is that of insulin resistance—a state in which, although insulin levels in the body are adequate, or even excessive, insulin is not being utilized well at the tissue level.

A lot of research is now being conducted on insulin resistance, and yet there is almost no open acknowledgment of the parallel phenomenon of thyroid-hormone resistance. If receptors for thyroid hormone are not soaking it up properly, then an individual will show the symptoms of hypothyroidism, including constant fatigue, *despite* adequate circulating levels of thyroid hormone. That is one big reason thyroid disease can be "hidden." Studies show that the use of small supplemental amounts of thyroid hormone—even in cases where blood tests show it to be adequate—can clear up symptoms. In one study of ten women with blood tests that indicated normal thyroid function and severe PMS, nine of the women reported dramatic improvement in their fatigue and other symptoms when given thyroid hormone.

Another problem that frequently crops up when doctors prescribe thyroid is that a patient doesn't respond as well as they had hoped. "Doctor, I'm still tired and depressed." The doctor may be more tempted to believe the blood test than the patient. However, if the patient is taking Synthroid, the synthetic thyroid most commonly prescribed, there may be another cause of continued fatigue. Synthroid is artificial T-4, which perfectly mimics the hormone secreted by the thyroid. However, the body needs to convert some of this T-4 into T-3, a different form. If the conversion is not complete or efficient, symptoms of thyroid deficiency can persist. An individual may actually need supplements of T-3 as well. Although useful tests have been designed to measure T-3, these T-3 levels only provide a partial clue to clinical response. As mentioned above, there may still be tissue resistance, and higher amounts of hormone may be required.

In borderline instances, I often add the TRH stimulation test. Half of the patients so tested end up needing thyroid medications. And at least nine out of ten of those patients are very appreciative because they benefit so hugely from the medication. An example of this was a patient of mine who had a borderline TSH test. Most endocrinologists would stop at that test, which was technically normal, but her symptoms were so pronounced (she was draggy, tired, and stiff in the morning, and she tended to gain weight) that I repeated the TSH test along with a TRH stimulation test. The next TSH was abnormal, but the real tie breaker was the TRH test. She clearly needed thyroid and felt much better once she began taking it.

Although I don't advocate dispensing thyroid hormone overzealously, endocrinologists today are perhaps overly stringent about dispensing the communion wafer of their profession. Also, they may not explain to patients that different types of thyroid are available, and that each type of thyroid has different effects (see box).

Hormones aren't the only answer to low thyroid. In some cases, I start treating subclinical low thyroid with the amino acid tyrosine, and essential vitamin and mineral co-factors for thyroid. Tyrosine is a building block for thyroid hormone.

Tyrosine turned out to be the "magic" solution for one of my patients. She was suffering from primary hypothyroidism—she was literally not producing enough hormone. Her major symptoms were fatigue and weight gain. But she was very reluctant to take thyroid medication, and I was equally concerned, because she suffered from a cardiac arrhythmia, and the hormone might have aggravated her heart problem. Her case was an extremely delicate one, and her cardiologist had recommended thyroid along with a heart drug known as Inderal. That meant she would be taking two powerful medications for the rest of her life.

Instead, I ordered blood tests that analyzed her nutritional status,

WHAT KIND OF THYROID MEDICATION SHOULD YOU TAKE?

▼

L-thyroxine (Synthroid) is most utilized by conventional endocrinologists. It is a synthetic analogue of thyroid hormone, containing the same amino-acid sequence. Doctors like it because Synthroid levels in the blood can be measured accurately by current tests, and so precise doses can be prescribed and regularly monitored.

Synthetic T-3 (Cytomel) is another medication currently available. The results can sometimes be remarkable. I've seen patients taking huge doses of Synthroid, or T-4, with little effect. Add T-3 and the response is immediate and pronounced.

Natural thyroid hormone is an extract of thyroid glands from beef or pork, available by prescription only. Endocrinologists are critical of it because it is difficult to standardize levels of natural extracts and so dose strength may vary minutely from batch to batch. It is also difficult to monitor response via blood levels. But clinically, my experience is that patients often respond best to this kind of supplementation, because the medication is in a natural form.

Glandulars, available in health-food stores across the country, supposedly contain extracts of thyroid gland without the hormone. Patients often resort to self-prescribed glandulars, but I don't recommend them. A recent study found that glandulars are actually *too* efficacious in some cases. Although the FDA has tried to eliminate active thyroid from these preparations, some brands seem to have sneaked through with actual hormone. One woman took glandulars and overdosed on them, developing hyperthyroidism.

Some chiropractors and naturopaths who advocate glandulars contend that even though in most cases they do not contain active hormone, they provide the body with a subtle signal to make more thyroid. I wonder. In my mind the use of glandulars is akin to the use of brain extracts to boost flagging memory. If the ingestion of freeze-dried brain actually had an impact on mental faculties, the French, with their large consumption of a national delicacy known as cerveaux (calves' brains), would be the most intelligent nation on earth, *n'est-ce pas?* (Many say they are!)

Dr. Royal Lee, in the 1930s and 1940s, was an ardent proponent of what was called "oral organotherapy," or the administration of small

(continued)

Tired All the Time

doses of glandular extracts, including liver, thyroid, adrenal, and ovary. A book by one of Lee's followers, Henry R. Harrower, entitled *Practical Organotherapy* ran to four editions with a total publication of 65,000. According to Harrower, glandular therapy provided a "homo-stimulative effect." "For many cases, judicious thyroid therapy seems to put the patient's own thyroid on a better plane of service," he contended.

and I found that she was abnormally low in tyrosine. When we supplemented this single amino acid, her function returned to normal. Other patients benefit from a cocktail of nutrients, including natural anti-inflammatory fatty acids, B vitamins that help transport oxygen inside the cells, and zinc and copper, both of which are important in helping the body make thyroid hormone.

Finally, and perhaps most important, if your TSH results are borderline, ask your doctor to repeat the test six months later. A borderline test can be a lab error, or it may mean you are moving toward an abnormal reading.

One proof of thyroid's profound impact on all aspects of health was a patient of mine I'll call John. I never would have suspected him of having low thyroid because he was extremely active physically. Only after a thirty-minute history did I learn that he was completely devastated by chronic fatigue.

John was a twenty-five-year-old man with a quiet, stoical personality—a man who rarely complained about anything. He ran six miles a day, and came to me because he'd recently noticed a swelling in his hands and feet, and a coarsening of his features. He also had experienced bizarre muscle aches and tingling in his fingers. His girlfriend was a medical technician, and over the last few months she had tested his blood in her laboratory at no cost. He brought me an array of tests with alarming abnormalities—from elevated liver enzymes to anemia to extremely high cholesterol. But, curiously, no thyroid tests were performed by these do-it-yourselfers. John's system was suppressed in so many ways that my mind leapt to one of the worst possibilities—

that he was suffering from AIDS. As calmly and evenly as possible, I inquired if he had ever used IV drugs, engaged in high-risk sexual activities, or had a blood transfusion. He had not. I was relieved.

To complete the array of tests, I ordered other blood tests, including thyroid function. The thyroid test was the clue—it came back with almost no thyroid hormone at all. He was so low in thyroid that it was only by sheer dint of his tremendous, almost Herculean determination that he was able to run. I found it remarkable. An ordinary individual with a thyroid that low would have been dragging from doctor to doctor with multiple complaints. (Interestingly, I recently learned that this man's complaint came under the rubric of Hoffman's syndrome, a now rare manifestation of severe hypothyroidism that results in muscle pain. This was my first encounter with the condition that bore my name!) John responded rapidly to thyroid, with a complete resolution of his symptoms. Even so, it took him almost a year to repair the damage done to his body.

When thyroid is low, it can have an extremely harmful effect on levels of other chemicals in the body. For instance, cholesterol can shoot up to dangerous levels. Thyroid is so effective at lowering cholesterol that one of the new drugs recently proposed to combat high cholesterol was a chemically modified version of thyroid—a version that doesn't dangerously speed up the heart rate but helps the body efficiently metabolize cholesterol.

One of my patients, Anna, a seventy-five-year-old woman, came in with an alarming cholesterol level of 385 and triglycerides of 550. She had followed a strict diet with no change in either reading, and so her doctor had urged her to take the latest lipid-lowering drug— but she'd experienced side effects of muscle pain and inflammation. Her coarse, thin white hair, dry and flaking skin, constant tiredness, croaky voice, and swollen hands and feet all suggested low thyroid. She was quite overweight despite her small intake of food. I ran the simplest thyroid test on her, and found that she was indeed hypothyroid. Because she was elderly, and I wanted to be careful not to strain her heart, I began her on a low dose, increasing the amount with each monthly visit. Within a year her cholesterol came down to 195, and her triglycerides plummeted to 120.

The punch line on Anna? One month she came back saying, "Doctor, I'm doing terrible. I'm feeling lousy. I'm almost back to where I was before I saw you." I looked at her lab tests and said, "I'm not surprised. Your cholesterol and triglycerides are up again. You must have gone off your diet."

"No, Dr. Hoffman, I'm eating even more carefully than ever. And I'm taking my thyroid as always."

I sat for a moment, musing. For some reason, a strange thought occurred to me. "What color is your thyroid pill?" I asked her, and when she said pink, I pulled out the *Physician's Desk Reference*, a huge, unwieldy tome that contains descriptions of every drug available and is the physician's surrogate Bible. "Is this it?" I asked, pointing to one of the pictures, and she nodded. I explained to Anna that the pharmacy had made a mistake on her latest prescription, and given her .025 milligrams instead of 0.25. "This month you've been taking one-tenth of what you need. No wonder you're feeling lousy." (This kind of mistake, unfortunately, is not rare. A recent study on patients discharged from the hospital with an average of three to four medications found that 50 percent were taking improper dosages, and 13 percent were victims of medication and prescription errors that were potentially dangerous.)

Although hypothyroidism is alarmingly common, I also see more and more exhausted patients who are actually hyperthyroid. Treatment for their problem is very different, for if ignored, excess thyroid hormone can cause serious and permanent health problems. One of my patients was a busy executive who had repeatedly ignored her doctors' pleas to let him treat her overactive thyroid. By the time she came to my office she had a dangerously large heart that fluttered in a rapid irregular rhythm. Though only forty-three, she was at risk for congestive heart failure and stroke. We treated her thyroid problem successfully.

Tests usually show quite clearly when a patient's thyroid is overactive. In that case, there are three options in conventional medicine: pills, radioactive iodine, or surgery. Medication can temporarily slow down the thyroid, but it may cause side effects, and its impact is often transient. Eventually the thyroid may simply gun its motor even higher.

Radioactive iodine is actually a medical cocktail that is swallowed. Because the thyroid instantly soaks up iodine, the radioactive material is concentrated there and does not circulate to other parts of the body. It kills some of the thyroid cells, leaving thyroid hormone at a lower level. The problem is that the precise dose of iodine to be given to an individual is practically impossible to determine. Often the patient is given too much and ends up hypothyroid—sometimes instantly, sometimes a year or two later.

The third and most invasive option, surgery, requires removing part of the gland under anesthesia in the hospital. Surgery may be chosen over radioactive iodine where the patient is pregnant.

I don't always recommend those three options. Though I differ radically from the conventional medical establishment in what I'm about to say, I do believe that borderline hyperthyroidism can sometimes be carefully watched, without the immediate use of medicines that permanently destroy thyroid function. Sometimes patients can use the thyroid "crisis" as an opportunity to learn stress reduction through meditation and relaxation. In my experience this will often gradually stabilize thyroid function in mild, borderline cases.

One of my patients, a hard-driving psychotherapist, had moderately elevated thyroid hormone levels. She was told of the need to use drugs or drink radioactive iodine. By cutting back her practice to twenty hours a week and taking up meditation and an organic, vegetarian diet, she normalized her thyroid in three months. She used the thyroid crisis as an impetus to balance her fragmented life. She heard, and heeded, her body's warning before it was too late.

The thyroid gland, a tiny powerhouse, is complex. But it is far simpler than another energy center in the body: the twin, almond-sized glands known as the adrenals.

I've seen many patients in my practice who are tired and vulnerable to infection because of weak adrenal response. They are like the white rabbits of a famous study that compared albino rabbits with a strain of wild rabbits. The albino rabbits were more susceptible to infection, extreme heat or cold, starvation, and even the effects of sudden fright. Their adrenal glands were also found by researchers to be smaller. The wild rabbits were wily, cagey, and hardy. My patients who suffer from adrenal "exhaustion" may have been born with smaller and weaker glands. They tend to have more allergies, blood-sugar abnormalities (adrenal cortisol counters the effect of insulin, and when cortisol is low, insulin may lower blood sugar excessively, causing patients to crave sugar).

When they are queried on their first visit, my "white rabbits" will say something like, "I've always been tired. I've had allergies as long as I can remember. I get four to six colds a year, and sometimes they turn into bronchitis."

Located just atop the kidneys, the adrenal glands have two parts: the cortex, which comes from the Latin word for tree bark, and the medulla. The cortex is the outer wrapping of the gland, and produces cortisol, a powerful anti-inflammatory hormone. The medulla, the inner part, pours out adrenaline and epinephrine, two of the most important hormones in the body. These two hormones govern the fight-or-flight response, and they are almost a direct extension of the nervous system.

Adrenaline and epinephrine are actually catecholamines, a class of chemicals that are associated with energy and euphoria; their effects are mimicked in drugs to treat depression. There is a theory that certain forms of depression are caused by a lack of these chemicals in the brain. Catecholamines are a double-edged sword, for they not only lift you up, they also make your heart race and your palms sweat.

When adrenal function is impaired or weak, a person may suffer from low blood sugar, low blood pressure, low body temperature, and a feeling of malaise and exhaustion. He may have very little endurance and find exercise strenuous. Adrenal exhaustion has recently been linked to chronic fatigue immune dysfunction syndrome. Patients with this condition may have less of an important hypothalamic hormone, CRH.

Little can be done to orchestrate the continual high-wire act of these hormones, which literally respond to the tiniest stimuli in the environment. Are you sitting down right now? Try standing up. Your adrenal glands just regulated an exquisite ballet of neurotransmitters and responded to pressure receptors so that the blood would not pool in your lower body and rush out of your head, causing you to faint.

The adrenal glands are absolutely instrumental in regulating how your nervous system responds to the stress of the world. How, then, can one possibly say to a patient, "Take some more Adrenalin. That will cure you"? The adrenal glands, unlike the thyroid, are not simply "high" or "low." People can become exhausted and weak, but no pill can offer the suppleness of response of the adrenals.

Nonetheless, these glands are so significant that we have countless medications to mimic or to counter their effects. Almost every asthma spray contains an adrenal-like hormone, whether it mimics adrenaline, epinephrine, or cortisol. Heart drugs that slow the heart rate and block the pain of angina contain "beta blockers" that stop the action of adrenaline and epinephrine.

As versatile as the adrenal medulla is, the adrenal cortex is even more so. It produces several hormones. The first are called mineralocorticoids, which govern the levels of sodium, potassium, and magnesium in the body. Sodium, on one hand, and magnesium and potassium, on the other, are on a kind of seesaw, powerfully affecting blood pressure as they are excreted or retained by the kidneys. Many blood-pressure drugs modulate the effect of mineralocorticoids.

The second hormone is one of the most wide-ranging and essential chemicals in the entire body. Called cortisol, it controls inflammation and impacts on everything from allergy to wound healing to countless diseases ranging from asthma to arthritis and lupus. The invention of a synthetic version of cortisol—called cortisone—was heralded as one of the most significant breakthroughs in twentieth-century medicine, on a par with the development of lifesaving antibiotics. Cortisone, embraced with worldwide fanfare and enthusiasm, was thought to be a panacea for a huge range of illnesses. Various versions of cortisone seemed to cure every type of inflammatory disease, reduced swelling of the brain after serious injury, and completely revolutionized the field of dermatology.

By now, we all know the dark aftermath of this drug—it gave a superb initial response with a terrible long-term price. On fifty milligrams of prednisone you feel great, even euphoric, as though your body were wrapped in cotton, but the price is enormous. The drug's side effects have included everything from diabetes to psychosis, unsightly ballooning of the cheeks and buffalo hump of the back, ulcers, bone thinning, and serious immune suppression. Worst of all, massive and prolonged doses of cortisone cause adrenal failure. The adrenals just stop manufacturing their own hormones, and sometimes that failure is irreversible.

Adrenal failure may be one reason that when a patient stops taking cortisone, he experiences a vicious "rebound" effect, where symptoms return with a vengeance. And yet, even now, cortisone is considered a virtual miracle worker in many situations: it can ease the unbearable pain of polymyositis or ulcerative colitis, save lives during acute allergic reactions, and help interrupt the inflammatory "spiral" of many conditions, putting them in remission or giving the body the rest it needs to regain balance and harmony. And in life-threatening conditions like the deadly pneumonia that AIDS patients often get, a dose of prednisone—a potent form of cortisone—can actually help the patient survive.

The conventional test for adrenal weakness is the ACTH stimulation test. ACTH is the pituitary hormone that signals the adrenal glands to release cortisol. A doctor can inject ACTH and measure the blood levels of cortisol both immediately and thirty minutes later. Weak adrenals fail the test. In my experience, however, this test misses many cases of adrenal weakness. I prefer to make a clinical diagnosis based on symptoms. I also measure blood and urine levels of a substance called DHEA, an adrenal hormone that enhances mood and immune response. DHEA has been found to help rheumatoid arthritis and other autoimmune diseases and in Europe is widely used to extend longevity, boost the immune system, and combat nervousness and exhaustion. If you suspect your adrenal function is low, you can ask your doctor to measure levels of DHEA.

For patients with weak adrenals, I find the best approach seems to be a mixture of herbs and nutrients that subtly mimic the effects of the adrenal glands. This may sound like pallid therapy at best, but these herbs can actually be quite potent. Every internist is aware of the danger of licorice consumption in patients with high blood pressure. That is because licorice has a powerful effect on the adrenal glands, slowing the breakdown of the mineralocorticoids, and causing the body to retain sodium. I had one eighty-year-old patient who drank so much licorice tea that his blood pressure soared from 90/60 to a dangerous 180/120 in a few months. In fact, licorice should only be taken under a doctor's supervision, and your blood pressure should be monitored. Licorice's active ingredient is glycyrrhizin, a plant hormone that enhances the action of the adrenal hormones.

Acupuncture and chiropractic can sometimes give the adrenals a much-needed boost as well. The adrenal glands are richly fed by nerves that connect to the spine, and by releasing blockages through these simple and effective techniques, the glands can be stimulated and strengthened.

From the standpoint of Oriental medicine, allergy and asthma are often treated by strengthening what is known as the "kidney" meridian—which translates, in Western terms, into the adrenal glands. People who are susceptible to infection or allergies are often told they have weak kidney chi (energy), and acupuncture points along the kidney meridian are stimulated. Sometimes a little fire is applied to the adrenals by application of heated incense, also known as moxibustion.

On occasion, very small doses of adrenal hormones may restore adrenal function. One apostle of this approach, William Jefferies (author of *Safe Uses of Cortisone*), believes that minute physiologic doses of these hormones can treat chronic fatigue, as well as allergies and other complaints. Though he's considered a maverick by most endocrinologists, he has documented successes, and his doses of hormones are so low that they're often unavailable in conventional pharmacies. As of this writing, his approach is considered controversial and may not be widely available.

Your Energy Plan

Suspect *hypothyroidism* if you are depressed, lethargic, easily chilled, overweight, or often tired, or if you suffer from dry skin, wake with muscle aches in the morning, have PMS, or get lots of colds and flu.

Take the Broda Barnes basal-body-temperature test. If it is positive, ask your doctor to test not only your thyroid function, but also your levels of thyroid-stimulating hormone. Ask him for a thyroid-releasing hormone (TRH) stimulation test. Also ask him to measure thyroid autoantibodies.

If you are hypothyroid, your doctor may put you on Synthroid. If it doesn't work, you may need synthetic T-3. Some doctors are willing to try natural thyroid hormone.

Suspect *hyperthyroidism* if you are hot, wired but tired, or unable to keep weight on, or suffer from insomnia, heart palpitations, a racing pulse, or fine hand tremors.

Tired All the Time

Ask your doctor to test your thyroid hormone levels. If they are borderline, try lifestyle changes for six months. If your test remains borderline or is high, discuss with your physician whether you want to try medication, radioactive iodine or, as a last resort, surgery. Be aware that no matter what the treatment, you may eventually become hypothyroid and need medication.

Suspect *weak adrenals* if you succumb often to allergies and infections, feel constantly exhausted, and suffer from low blood sugar and low blood pressure. Ask your doctor to measure not only cortisol with the ACTH stimulation test but DHEA as well. If your adrenal response is weak, try acupuncture, chiropractic, meditation, and herbs that boost the adrenal glands, including licorice. Learn to relax!

4

SEX AND FATIGUE

▼

A new disease has emerged on the American medical landscape. It is called by the ominous name of "ovarian failure." Its symptoms are constant fatigue, moodiness, and hot flashes. The "drug" used to combat this disease is the fourth-best-selling medication in the United States: Premarin, a form of estrogen.

That is, in essence, what some of my colleagues in the field of gynecology are saying. Many doctors automatically prescribe estrogen-replacement therapy to "ease" the "failure" and energy loss of menopause.

I differ from doctors who believe we can simply replenish hormones and offer our patients a veritable fountain of youth. Although hormone-replacement therapy is sometimes necessary and beneficial, it should not be given automatically. The side effects of excess estrogen can be debilitating. One of my patients recently came to see me because she had experienced heavy menstrual bleeding at age fifty-four, after menopause. The bleeding was in response to Premarin, and was so profuse that she had become anemic. Her doctor had to administer another drug to reduce the bleeding, and she finally came to me seeking an alternative.

A huge number of my patients come to me because of constant fatigue and discomfort linked to hormonal fluctuations—whether they are due to menopause or PMS. This is actually fortunate, because hormonal imbalances often respond beautifully to a nutritional approach.

Why have we come to regard a natural, biological transition as a state of disease? A well-nourished and well-exercised body adjusts to the changes of menopause. Many women in the world are in a productive, stable, and highly energized menopause. Think, for instance, of rural China, where elderly peasant women labor in the fields daily.

Tired All the Time

In fact, rural China is known for its athletic competitions among the revered elderly: women in their seventies race across a field balancing large wooden buckets of water on their heads. The image may seem comical, but it really illustrates the hale and hearty nature of older women in societies other than our own.

Similarly, a healthy woman does not have to endure the ups and downs of PMS—another so-called hormonal "disease" of modern times. There is no doubt that hormones are powerfully linked to fatigue—but it is also true that hormones can be calibrated and balanced through natural means. I've seen it in my own patients countless times.

How is fatigue linked to hormones? There are two times in a woman's life when, because of female hormones, she may experience profound and even debilitating fatigue. Those times are just before the first onset of menstruation and at menopause. Both are periods of abrupt hormonal transition, and the key word here *is* transition. It is not the presence or absence of hormones that is exhausting to the body. It's the roller-coaster hormonal changes that stress your system and cause fatigue.

That's one reason blood tests don't help. If you have PMS, you can go to your doctor, tell her you think you have a hormone problem, and ask for blood tests. They will measure the absolute levels of hormones in your blood. But hormones go up and down like the Dow Jones average, and it's not the absolute levels that cause the blues so much as their delicate and ever-changing balance. Fatigue, in fact, is one of the first and most common responses to hormonal fluctuations.

To get an idea of the enormous complexity and delicacy of the endocrine system—and how easily it can be thrown off balance by a single feedback error—consider the typical hormonal changes that occur in the average woman's menstrual cycle (opposite page).

Do you wonder if you may be suffering from PMS-type hormonal blues? If so, answer the following questions:

1. Is your fatigue cyclical? Do you notice that it is worse before your period and improves afterward?

2. How much weight do you gain before your period? If it is more than five pounds, your hormonal changes probably have a profound impact on how you feel, and your brain is probably exposed to chemical changes that affect you adversely.

Sex and Fatigue

HORMONAL CHANGES IN THE MENSTRUAL CYCLE

▼

During the active reproductive part of a woman's life, all the sex hormones are constantly circulating at baseline levels. At the same time, there are minute fluctuations in these levels that powerfully affect a woman's body. There are three glands that do a kind of chemical dance together during the menstrual cycle: the pituitary, the hypothalamus, and the ovaries. What happens is this:

The *hypothalamus*, which is seated in an evolutionarily ancient part of the brain called the limbic system, monitors the levels of hormones produced by the ovaries. It also responds to external events, such as stress or sexual attraction, which is why women's menstrual cycles are sometimes susceptible to emotional influences. Stress or bereavement may cause them to cease altogether, or a new romantic involvement may cause irregular menses to normalize.

When the level of estrogen drops below a certain level, the hypothalamus sends out a hormone called GnRH (gonadotropin-releasing hormone). This hormone stimulates the pituitary, which then releases a hormone called FSH (follicle-stimulating hormone). FSH stimulates the ovary, and between ten and twenty of the ovary's follicles start to mature. As they mature, the follicles release more estrogen. This estrogen stimulates the lining of the uterus, which begins to grow in preparation for a fertilized egg. (Inside each follicle is an egg.)

Only one of the follicles matures fully. The others start to atrophy. The mature follicle continues to secrete estrogen, which stimulates the pituitary to release large amounts of FSH and another hormone, LH (luteinizing hormone). The combination of FSH and LH, in turn, stimulates the follicle, which releases its precious egg. At the same time, the follicle itself begins to secrete huge amounts of progesterone and far less estrogen. The name of the follicle in this stage is *corpus luteum*.

The progesterone stimulates the uterine lining and prepares it to receive and nourish the fertilized egg. If the egg is indeed fertilized, the corpus luteum continues to secrete hormones during the entire pregnancy. It is "told" to do this by a hormone called HCG (human chorionic gonadotropin), which is secreted by the placenta, the sac that wraps the embryo. If, however, the egg is not fertilized, the corpus luteum begins to disintegrate. It no longer releases hormones. The diminishing levels of estrogen and progesterone fail to nourish the uterine lining, and so it begins to slough off. The process is known as menstruation. And then the complex ballet begins again.

3. Do you experience extreme cravings for sugary or spicy foods or chocolate? A day or two of craving is probably normal, but if you have profound cravings that last for a week or more, you are probably suffering from PMS.

4. Do other women in the family (your mother, sister, or daughter) suffer similar symptoms?

5. Are you profoundly sensitive to the birth-control pill? Did it cause you to develop side effects such as migraines or breast tenderness?

If you answered yes to any of the above questions, suspect a hormonal imbalance as a significant cause of your fatigue.

Once you've ascertained that PMS may indeed be a cause of your tiredness, you need to determine what type of PMS you may be suffering from. According to Guy Abraham, a pioneering physician who researched it for over a decade, premenstrual syndrome is not just one condition but four. However, many patients experience more than one of the following types of premenstrual tension (PMT). In fact, about 75 percent of all PMS patients have PMT-A, 60 percent have PMT-H, 40 percent have PMT-C, and 30 percent have PMT-D. Each type of PMS seems due to a specific hormonal imbalance. Therefore, Dr. Abraham has formulated a vitamin and mineral supplement called OptiVite, which contains a balance of nutrients known to be helpful in premenstrual syndrome.

Look at the four types of PMS outlined on the opposite page and see if any of the symptoms are familiar.

After decades of the intricate monthly ballet of menstruation, menopause begins. I liken this time to the body's version of the *1812 Overture*—hormonal production soars, sputters, and plummets. Counterregulatory hormones skyrocket in an effort to maintain balance. These precipitous hormone highs and lows exhaust the body, producing continual withdrawal reactions and affecting all the tissues.

Whether I am treating a woman for fatigue related to PMS or menopause, my most powerful weapon is diet. Diet can be amazingly effective in reducing the level of excess hormones. Here are my most common dietary rules:

1. Reduce animal fat. That is because of one important component of inflammation: prostaglandins. These potent, hormonelike chemicals

THE FOUR TYPES OF PREMENSTRUAL SYNDROME

▼

PMT-A (Anxiety), the most common, is characterized by nervous tension, mood swings, irritability, anxiety, and insomnia. Hormonally, blood levels of estrogen are high, while progesterone is low. Patients tend to consume excess dairy products and refined sugars.

(One of my favorite tests for PMT-A is to ask a patient facetiously, "Do you break down in tears when you see a long-distance phone ad?" I was caught short by the answer to this question once when I found out my patient actually worked in the ad agency that produced those ads. "I don't cry at my own ads," was her response, "but I do cry at the other ones.")

Treatment: In double-blind studies, vitamin B6, in doses of 200–800 mg daily, has been shown to reduce estrogen and increase progesterone, thus easing symptoms.

PMT-H (Hyperhydration), the second most common, is characterized by weight gain; swelling of hands, feet, and ankles; breast tenderness; and bloating of the stomach. Water and salt are retained.

Treatment: Vitamin B6 and vitamin E have both been shown to help. Sodium should be limited.

PMT-C (Craving) is characterized by fatigue, headaches, a craving for sweets, increased appetite, a pounding heart, and dizziness or fainting. It is associated with low blood levels of magnesium, and also of one of the "good" anti-inflammatory prostaglandins.

Treatment: Supplements of magnesium, chromium, and GLA (gamma linolenic acid, which will be discussed later in this chapter) help improve symptoms.

PMT-D (Depression) is the least common but most dangerous, because suicide is most frequent in this group. It is characterized by depression, forgetfulness, crying, insomnia, and confusion. In PMT-D, the levels of progesterone are higher than normal at mid-month, while estrogen is lower, and in some cases, the levels of adrenal androgens are also higher.

Treatment: Herbs with weak estrogenlike hormones can help balance the body.

help control inflammation in the body, and it is thought that they may be linked to the symptoms caused by female hormonal imbalance. Some prostaglandins cause inflammation, while others reduce it. The ingredients in over-the-counter medicines like aspirin actually help reduce inflammation by blocking the action of "bad" prostaglandins—as well as good.

What is the link to animal fat? The body uses animal fat to make inflammatory prostaglandins. Cutting down on meat and fatty dairy products can sometimes do wonders for PMS.

2. Bolster "good," anti-inflammatory prostaglandins by adding their nutritional building blocks to your diet. In particular, supplement your diet with GLA, found in evening primrose oil, borage oil, and black currant-seed oil. These can be bought in health-food stores.

3. Eat a diet low in sugar and refined carbohydrates. Patients suffering from premenstrual symptoms tend to have diets high in these foods. A low-sugar diet tends to reduce blood-sugar swings, which can intensify symptoms. During episodes of PMS, patients often break out into a sweat during hypoglycemic episodes, mimicking the flushes and sweats of menopause. Women may even be more predisposed to hypoglycemia at certain times of the month. Avoid alcohol, which can disrupt the metabolism of the "good" prostaglandins.

4. Slowly add fiber to your diet. Fiber helps dietary sugar to be released over time, and for sufferers of PMS, it can literally soak up excess estrogen. Women on high-fiber vegetarian diets maintain more moderate estrogen levels in their bodies and suffer less PMS. They also suffer fewer hormonally related cancers (breast, uterus, and possibly ovary). Cruciferous vegetables, such as broccoli, cabbage, and brussels sprouts, have been proved to regulate levels of estradiol, one of the most powerful estrogens in your body. If your problem is excess estrogen related to PMS, these vegetables may be helpful.

5. Add herbs and foods that have plant hormones. Plant hormones are like weak versions of human hormones, and sometimes, rather than boosting overall hormone levels, they can actually fill the hormone receptors in the body, so that you are less affected by your own excess hormones. Or, if you are depleted in hormones, they can boost your own system.

Herbs like black cohosh, chasteberry, licorice, ginseng, and others contain natural estrogens. The wild yam contains a natural building block for progesterone, and is available from nutritionists and in some health-food stores as an extract in a cream called Pro-Gest. Some herbalists also make powdered extracts of the yam. Other studies show that a traditional Japanese diet tends to prevent premenstrual tension and hormonally linked cancers, and one reason may be because of the plant estrogens in soybean, which seem to block receptors for potent human estrogens.

The best way to take herbs is to start with low doses and build slowly until they improve your well-being. You may have to experiment to find the particular herbs to which your body is most responsive.

6. Add nutritional supplements. Many women are driven by a tremendous craving for chocolate before their periods. Cocoa is known to be one of the richest sources of magnesium. Magnesium is often depleted in patients suffering from PMS. It's a smooth-muscle relaxer, and tends to be calming. Calcium is also beneficial, because it is a messenger chemical for almost every energy reaction in the body. For women exhausted by the changes of menopause, natural supplements like the mineral boron can jump-start the body's flagging production of estrogen. Vitamin B6 may act like a natural diuretic, counteracting water retention.

7. Take herbs that boost the liver, such as dandelion and milk thistle. The liver is the organ that detoxifies estrogen in the body, and when it is sluggish or overloaded with other toxins, it may not do the job as well.

One of the most dramatic and beneficial treatments for extreme PMS is something called the Meyers' cocktail. It was named after its inventor, John Meyers of Baltimore, who developed a devoted following of women patients who decades ago trekked monthly to his office for an intravenous drip of nutrients and vitamins. The Meyers' cocktail contains a PMS formulation of magnesium, calcium, vitamin C, and B vitamins, all of which drip directly into the bloodstream, where they can rush instantly to vulnerable organs.

This cocktail worked when nothing else would for Nancy, a nurse who came to see me because before her period she went into such a deep depression and felt so fatigued she was unable to function. She could only work as a part-time per-diem nurse because of these monthly black moods and exhaustion. She had been treated unsuccessfully with antidepressants. I suggested dietary change and a Meyers' cocktail twice a week. As her symptoms improved over time, she was able to reduce her intravenous drips to once a month. Today she has a full-time job as a nursing supervisor.

Unfortunately, intravenous drips are not available from most doctors in the country. Nonetheless, many nutritionally oriented physicians do offer this approach, and if it's available to you it's worth trying. Contact either the American College for Advancement in Medicine (714-583-7666, in Laguna Hills, California) or the American Academy of Environmental Medicine (303-622-9755, in Denver, Colorado) for referrals to physicians in your area.

Perhaps the most overlooked way to balance your body's hormones is through the simple act of exercise. Exercise is an important PMS fighter, because it lowers estrogen levels (sometimes so dramatically that some marathoners stop having periods).

Acupuncture can also help revitalize the fatigued victim of PMS and menopause. In Chinese medicine, acupuncture has long been used for gynecologic problems. Acupuncture directed to the reproductive system may actually alter the release of estrogen, cortisol, and other hormones. One ingenious double-blind study, sponsored by the Kaiser Foundation Research Institute several years ago, examined women suffering from menstrual pain. Eleven women were given "real" acupuncture treatment at appropriate acupuncture sites. A second group of eleven women were given "placebo" acupuncture at sites that were random. A third group of eleven women was followed without any intervention. Of the "real" acupuncture group, 10 improved (90.9 percent). Of the "placebo" group, 4 improved (36.4 percent). Of the control group, 2 improved (18.2 percent). Although the sample was small, the results are intriguing.

There is also a controversial new approach to the bleak exhaustion that can accompany PMS and menopause. It focuses on the fact that many women may be hypersensitive to their own hormones. Cases have been documented where women experienced monthly anaphylaxis—a severe and even life-threatening allergic reaction where the throat closes, the body swells with hives, and the patient ends up in the emergency room. This kind of allergic reaction is well known as a response to bee stings—but on rare occasions, women have experienced it premenstrually in reaction to their own hormones. One pioneering physician, Carlton Lee, proposed that many women may be allergically sensitive to their own hormones, and this hypersensitivity may cause symptoms when the hormones swing out of balance. This can happen before the period or during menopause.

If Dr. Lee's theory is true, women can receive "allergy" neutralization for their hormones, just as typical hay-fever sufferers receive allergy shots for pollen. In my practice, I've seen many women regain their energy and equilibrium after receiving neutralization for estrogen, progesterone, and some of the mid-cycle hormones that stimulate the ovaries. One woman, Sophie, was already sixty, and her hot flashes, moodiness, and fatigue had dragged on for years—it seemed as if she had never recovered from menopause. Dietary changes hadn't helped much. We challenged her with minute amounts of several hormones and found she had a profound hypersensitivity. We could literally turn her symptoms on and off at will!

Whenever we talk about the endocrine system and fatigue, women come to mind. Women are far more susceptible than men to endocrine causes of fatigue—whether through low thyroid or menstrual problems. In fact, the symptoms of PMS and hypothyroidism are strikingly similar: weight gain, lethargy, irritability, moodiness, low body temperature, and anxiety. In one interesting study published in the *New England Journal of Medicine*, fifty-four women with PMS were studied, and 94 percent were found to have one or more laboratory indications of thyroid dysfunction. An astonishing 31 percent had a severe thyroid disorder. When patients were treated with synthetic thyroid hormone, their PMS symptoms cleared up.

But hormonally based fatigue can and does strike men as well, and too often it is overlooked by physicians. This kind of exhaustion is usually linked to the male hormone testosterone. Men don't undergo a decisive, life-altering event like menopause. Their hormones slowly, insidiously decline. In some cases, abnormally low testosterone can cause debilitating fatigue and a low libido. One such patient, Tom, came in suffering from an autoimmune disease similar to lupus. He had serious lung problems and was so depressed and hopeless about his condition that he failed to keep his next appointment. Looking at his lab results, however, I saw how low his testosterone was and thought I could help him. I called him up two months after his initial visit and urged him to come in.

"My life is over," he told me. "What's the point?"

I convinced him to come in and prescribed a battery of anti-inflammatory nutrients, along with lifestyle changes. I also prescribed testosterone, and he is now one of my biggest success stories: his "lust" for life has literally returned.

Your Energy Plan

FOR PMS:

Take the PMS Quiz. If you believe you are suffering from PMS, ascertain which type (or types) you suffer from, and note which supplements (B6, magnesium, GLA) you should emphasize.

Follow the general dietary rules for hormonal imbalance:

• Cut down on dairy and animal protein to reduce levels of inflammatory prostaglandins.

• Supplement your diet with GLA.

• Add fiber. If your problem is excess estrogen, emphasize cruciferous vegetables like broccoli, cabbage, and brussels sprouts.

• Reduce sugar in your diet. Low blood sugar can exacerbate hormone blues.

• Add herbs with weak plant hormones that mimic human hormones: Dong Quai, angelica, black cohosh, chasteberry, licorice, wild yam, and ginseng.

• Start an exercise program to balance hormones, blood sugar, and energy levels.

• Boost liver function with herbs like dandelion and milk thistle and "lipotropic" nutrients like choline, inositol, and the amino acid methionine.

• Try acupuncture.

• If you have access to a physician who is willing to give you an intravenous Meyers' cocktail, consider trying it.

• Work with an allergist who is willing to neutralize your reactions to your own hormones. For a listing, contact the American Academy of Environmental Medicine.

FOR MENOPAUSE:

• Try acupuncture.
• Add herbs with estrogenlike properties. Add boron, a trace mineral that boosts your natural levels of estrogen, and magnesium, vitamin E, and gamma linolenic acid, which can be found in borage oil, blackcurrant-seed oil, and evening primrose oil.
• Reduce dietary sugar.
• Try neutralization shots with an environmental physician.
• Exercise.

FOR MEN ONLY:

• Ask your doctor to check your testosterone level. In the event that it is low, replacement hormone may revitalize you.

5

DO YOU HAVE A SUGAR DISEASE?

Thyroid disease may be rampant, and adrenal exhaustion may be a common sign of stress, but there is a third, remarkable hormone that is a keystone of health and energy: insulin. And as you may have suspected, sugar consumption is so widespread in this country that countless Americans suffer from insulin surges that ultimately damage their health and lead to hypoglycemia, diabetes, heart disease, and chronic tiredness. Balancing your blood sugar—and your insulin levels—is an important part of regaining energy and health.

Surprising as it sounds, sugar is more potent than many drugs. Sugar was once a luxury so rare it was offered as a sacrifice to the gods. A Hindu religious pamphlet from about 500 A.D. tells of the rolling of balls of sugar. In seventh-century Persia, when epidemics plagued the land, a piece of sugar was considered a precious miracle drug. By the year 1100, when sugar finally reached England, a pound cost the equivalent of a year's salary. But by 1700, Britain was importing 20 million pounds of sugar a year. Today each person in the United States consumes an average of 125 pounds of refined sugar a year.

Sugar is an essential component of health and balance: when blood sugar is low, the body's cells—particularly the brain cells—are starved. To maintain optimal health, the body needs to keep a constant balance between glucose and oxygen in the bloodstream. What happens when you eat refined sugar, also known as sucrose? Unlike complex carbohydrates, which require time to be broken down, sucrose is quickly absorbed into the blood, upsetting the precise balance between insulin and glucose. Balance is destroyed. The body goes into crisis. Here is what happens:

Blood glucose soars, and we feel a temporary lift. At the same time, hormones pour out from the adrenal glands and sound the call to arms. Insulin bursts from the pancreas and helps hold down the glucose level in the blood. Usually, because this happens under "emergency" conditions, the blood glucose soon crashes, and a second crisis occurs. We feel exhausted, listless, and irritable. The cells of the brain, in particular, depend completely upon moment-to-moment blood-sugar nourishment—and mood swings due to sugar highs and lows can result. (In fact, many patients who suffer from frequent panic attacks are hypoglycemic—and blood sugar is the key to controlling the anxiety triggered by sugar surges and crashes.) The pancreas has to shut down, and new adrenal hormones pour out to help raise the blood glucose.

In sum, sugar takes a tremendous toll on your body's metabolic machinery by triggering fatiguing surges of insulin and counterregulatory stress hormones. If you doubt that, all you'd have to do is watch a patient relaxing and reading magazines in a comfortable, oversized leather chair in my laboratory while he or she is being given a glucose-tolerance test. The erratic fluctuations in blood sugar require such a Herculean effort on the part of the body—which continually tries to pour out regulatory and counterregulatory hormones—that patients often describe the experience as "exhausting." Usually I intervene and give them a glass of orange juice before they leave the office. Any patient who has been through this experience finally gets the message about sugar. It is as if the knowledge is finally imprinted in the patient's neural circuitry.

LOW BLOOD SUGAR AND ADRENAL FUNCTION

▼

After years on a sugar roller coaster, the adrenals can become damaged and worn out. One fascinating study recently hinted at a reason why: when rats were injected with massive doses of insulin in order to force them into a state of hypoglycemia, their adrenals almost instantly lost half of their vitamin C content. Vitamin C is crucial to adrenal function, and it may be that low blood sugar leaches this important nutrient from the adrenals. In fact, hypoglycemia is known in biology experiments to be as potent a stress on animals as shock, or being thrown into an icy pool and forced to swim.

Do You Have a Sugar Disease?

Why do I call sugar craving a disease? Excess sugar consumption is one of the major causes of fatigue, a situation still largely unrecognized by medicine. That is one reason I find it amazing that sugar is so often equated with fuel, because it is a fuel ill suited to the human body. The combination of a craving for sweets plus low blood sugar not only can tire you out but can trigger a disease process that spans decades. An individual may succumb to sugar cravings a million times in the course of a lifetime, generating a staggering overproduction of insulin, and often leading to a condition now known as "syndrome X," which is a precursor of heart disease and diabetes. In fact, the term "sugar disease" is a convenient catchall for a host of modern conditions that result from an unbridled intake of sugar or refined carbohydrates. Its three cardinal forms are:

1. hypoglycemia
2. syndrome X
3. diabetes

The three syndromes are often linked, and all three can cause profound, constant fatigue. I often have a feeling of eerie prescience about some of my patients with sugar disease. I've seen too many lean twenty-year-olds with hypoglycemia, slightly chubby thirty-year-olds with impaired glucose tolerance (and often real diabetes during pregnancy, which then recedes after childbirth), and middle-aged patients who gain weight and come down with full-blown diabetes and heart disease. It's almost as if this procession of patients at different ages together form one archetypal patient slowly succumbing to sugar disease.

Hypoglycemia

We are a society in love with carbohydrates. And though we talk up fiber, what is often palmed off as a high-fiber food is a commercial brown bread made of whole-wheat flour along with white flour, in a wrapper with a log cabin on the front—a far cry from the true fiber intake of our ancestors. In fact, the beautiful Adirondack Mountains of New York are named after an old Indian tribe called the Adirondacks, which translates as "bark eaters." These Indians had a late-winter habit of stripping bark from trees and eating it as a hedge against starvation. How's that for high fiber? Our stoutest whole-grain bread is like breakfast pastry by comparison.

The patient of mine who convinced me, once and for all, of the harm that sugar can cause used to be nicknamed Cookie by her colleagues at the office. She even called herself the Cookie Monster. She couldn't stop eating cookies, and she was exhausted beyond belief. Her exhaustion remitted completely when she was put on a diet of complex carbohydrates, protein at short intervals throughout the day to normalize her blood sugar, and nutritional supplements.

In essence, hypoglycemia is low blood sugar. If you ask a conventional physician, hypoglycemia is a rare, practically nonexistent malady. The next time you go to a doctor, try asking him or her if the symptoms you experience are due to hypoglycemia. You will undoubtedly evoke a bemused look, perhaps an angry one, or even a referral to a psychiatrist. Or perhaps your doctor will reluctantly perform a glucose-tolerance test to humor you. Don't bother. Glucose-tolerance tests, as performed conventionally, are biased to corroborate the point your doctor wants to make: you never had hypoglycemia in the first place!

But the truth is that hypoglycemia is far more prevalent than we're led to believe. Studies show that even in its full-blown form, it is often missed as a diagnosis: of thirty-nine patients who had tumors in the pancreas, a rare condition causing profound hypoglycemia, eight were first diagnosed with epilepsy or neurosis. That is not surprising, considering the following array of symptoms caused by hypoglycemia: spaciness, fatigue, mood changes, PMS, sugar craving, headaches, difficulty focusing the eyes, tremors, temperamental outbursts, depression, excessive sweating, hot flashes, palpitations, cold extremities, abdominal pain, panic attacks.

With such a laundry list of vague and seemingly subjective attributions, no wonder conventional doctors take a dim view of this condition. But hypoglycemia is nonetheless real.

Why so many symptoms? To learn the answer, we have to explore the physiology of low blood sugar.

The body is designed to digest, assimilate, and utilize three primary nutrients: proteins, fats, and carbohydrates. Proteins and fats can be used for energy, but their conversion to usable forms is gradual, not immediate. That is why athletes on low-carbohydrate diets often suffer an energy "brownout"—they perform less well than when provided with fuel in the readily usable form of carbohydrates.

Carbohydrates are all more or less readily digested into sugar. Their rate of conversion to sugar depends on their complexity. Complex carbohydrates, like beans, provide a slow time release of the sugar they contain in complex molecules of starch with fiber. The presence of natural "starch blockers" in beans further slows the sugar-liberation process.

On the other hand, sugars and refined carbohydrates provide a rapid sugar fix. This results in an immediate, pleasant sense of gratification—sometimes associated with mild drowsiness—the familiar sugar high. But then, in response, the body calls upon its insulin reserves, generated in the pancreas, to lower the blood sugar. This often happens precipitously. "What goes up must come down"—sometimes with crashing rapidity.

Experiments have now confirmed what the hypoglycemic experiences. Low blood sugar triggers hunger—especially carbohydrate craving. In addition, the brain is starved for its preferred fuel—glucose. At rest, the brain consumes one-third of the body's total glucose requirement. The brain is a hungry, rapidly metabolizing organ—and fuel shortages here create problems in concentration, memory, and mood.

Low blood sugar so profoundly affects the body it can even result in a state that looks like catatonic schizophrenia—a report in the journal *Emergency Medicine* told of a patient who was brought unconscious to the hospital one morning. The doctor lifted the patient's arm up in the air, walked out of the room, and came back to find the arm still lifted, a classic symptom of schizophrenia. The patient's temperature was only 94 degrees. When he was given intravenous glucose, however, he woke up and explained that he was a diabetic and had taken his morning insulin but had not eaten. As a result, his blood sugar had plummeted, resulting in hypoglycemia so severe he lost touch with reality.

But perhaps most important, low blood sugar triggers an outpouring of counterregulatory hormones (catecholamines), mostly from the adrenals. These hormones oppose the action of insulin and push blood sugar back up. Unfortunately for the hypoglycemic, these "rescue" hormones are the very same ones that produce the adrenaline rush of a fight-or-flight reaction. The results are symptoms like palpitations, sweaty palms, nervousness, tremor, and sometimes even severe panic attacks, followed by tremendous fatigue.

What can you do if you fear you suffer from blood-sugar swings? The best idea is to test yourself by going off sugar completely. Ultimately, it's the only way that works. The results can seem quite disastrous at first. Many of my patients report a week or more of severe fatigue and almost supernatural cravings for sugar. They may be unable to concentrate and may feel fidgety, irritable, and deeply depressed. I'm often inundated with phone calls in that first week. I'm also amazed at how resourceful some of my patients can be at finding ways to sneak sugar into their diet. "Gee, doc," a patient will say, catching me in the hall, "I just found something in the health-food store called barley malt. And rice syrup. Those are okay, aren't they?" Actually, they're not. They are simply alternative forms of sugar.

I don't relish being a food policeman, but this period of withdrawal is necessary. Sugar is a form of addiction. In fact, I have a hunch that the same hereditary susceptibility that leads to alcoholism may be involved in sugar addiction. Virtually all recovered alcoholics are "carboholics." One study in the *American Journal of Clinical Nutrition* found that alcoholics don't consume much sugar until they withdraw from alcohol. Most alcohols are not high in sugar and don't trigger actual blood-sugar surges. I suspect that alcohol and sugar have similarly intoxicating effects on brain cells and that perhaps they impact brain chemistry in similar ways. Many of my patients who are "carboholics" have a family history of alcoholism. "I don't drink any alcohol, Dr. Hoffman. I've had a family tragedy around that." And yet they are addicted to sugar.

People actually use sugar as medicine. And it may indeed be just that, according to remarkable studies by Judith and Richard Wurtman of MIT, as well as other nutrition researchers. Sugar tends to change the way the blood-brain barrier selects appropriate amino-acid building blocks of brain chemicals. Carbohydrate intake promotes uptake of the amino acid tryptophan, which is the building block for a brain chemical called serotonin. Serotonin is a proven tranquilizer. Certain individuals suffer major depression as a result of low levels of serotonin in the brain, and they can be enormously helped by drugs like Prozac, which promote high levels of serotonin.

Because sugar might combat depression, some researchers suggest using sugary snacks to "feed" the brain. I disagree. My belief is that sugar perpetuates a cycle of craving and bingeing. I would use tryptophan (which was formerly a treatment for depression, particularly in Great Britain), but because of a well-publicized incident of tryptophan contamination that resulted in tragic poisoning, this amino acid is not available.

The best answer, then, is to switch to a diet of protein and complex carbohydrates, which provide the body with slowly released and steady levels of sugar.

SUGAR CONTENT OF COMMON FOODS
Grams of Sugar per 100 Grams of Food

Fruit		Vegetable		Other	
Raisins	64	Sweet potato	9	Jam	69
Dates	64	Carrot	9	Chocolate	56–65
Banana	16	Onion	5	Iced cake	54
Apricot	16	Leeks	4	Plain cake	32
Grape	15	Peas	4	Ice cream	23
Apple	12	Tomato	3	Coca-Cola	11
Pineapple	12	Pumpkin	3	Corn flakes	7
Pear	11	Cabbage	2		
Orange	9	Lentils	1		

Adapted from the *International Clinical Nutrition Review,* January 1991

Syndrome X

Heart disease is not simply limited to the heart, for the heart pumps our lifeblood through the entire body, nourishing every single cell. If enough blood can't reach the cells, they will always be partially starved. The result: we seem sapped of life, tired all the time.

Our national call to arms against fat should be matched with a call to arms against sugar—and then we would truly see a remarkable drop in heart disease. Physicians are becoming more aware of nutrition lately, but it often seems as if their only advice for preventing heart disease is to avoid cholesterol and saturated fat. Syndrome X explains why that advice may not be enough—and why some patients on a "prudent" diet go on to develop heart disease without apparent cause.

You may be wondering what all this talk about sugar has to do with exhaustion. People with syndrome X are beset with an energy crisis. Their metabolism is at war with itself—too much high-energy food is stored as fat and too little is efficiently liberated as energy.

Syndrome X is a hot new concept on the cutting edge of medical research these days, but just like the importance of cholesterol a decade or so ago, its importance hasn't yet trickled down to the level of most frontline care deliverers. The syndrome X model envisions not just excess fat and cholesterol but also plentiful carbohydrates—especially the refined ones—as keys to the process of arteriosclerosis.

How could that be? Remember the insulin surge we get with sugar intake? Replicate that surge many thousands of times over the course of a lifetime and you end up with an overly sensitive insulin trigger and chronically elevated insulin. Why is that bad?

Consider these adverse effects of too much insulin:

1. weight gain, especially around the midsection
2. elevated blood pressure
3. elevated cholesterol and triglycerides
4. increased deposits of plaque in the arterial walls
5. immune suppression
6. insulin resistance

It's the latter that leads to the most common form of diabetes we see in the industrialized world: adult-onset diabetes. You can be a diabetic even when you have high levels of insulin in your body. In fact, this is a common occurrence in adult-onset non–insulin-dependent diabetes. Your insulin receptors, after years of being bombarded with signals from insulin, become less sensitive. More and more insulin is required to get the job done, until no amount will successfully lower blood sugar. The analogy is the boy who cried wolf so often that when the wolf actually appeared, nobody believed him. Diabetes is triggered by a diet high in sugar, and during the early stages there may be no detectable changes in blood sugar—although high levels of insulin may be discovered on a glucose/insulin-tolerance test.

Small wonder, then, that syndrome X leads to heart disease and may, in fact, be *the most prevalent cause of degenerative disease and premature death in modern society*.

How can you tell if you have syndrome X? A variation on the standard glucose-tolerance test, called the glucose/insulin-tolerance test (see below), will confirm it, but there are easier ways to tell:

1. An elevation of your triglycerides on a fasting blood test should alert your doctor to the fact that you're prone to syndrome X.

2. Even simpler, a quick tape measurement of waist and hips will yield a "waist-to-hip ratio." Waist divided by hip circumference in men should be no greater than 1.0; in women, no greater than 0.8. If it's greater, you've got the "central adiposity" that's a hallmark of syndrome X.

One patient of mine was a stock-market executive in his mid-thirties who had a familial tendency to high cholesterol. He came to me complaining of fatigue, and mentioned that his doctor was advocating a new cholesterol-lowering drug. He was a lean man, but with a small abdominal pouch—a tipoff for syndrome X. His father had suffered a heart attack at age fifty-eight, his mother had diabetes, and his brother had already undergone bypass surgery at forty-four. My patient was frankly worried. He was so tired every afternoon he consumed several "energy" bars and kept a mini-refrigerator in his office stocked with orange and apple juice. His afternoon carbohydrate binges staved off episodes of exhaustion; he sometimes just had to put his head on his desk and sleep.

When I asked about his diet he told me proudly how he'd eliminated breakfasts of sausage and scrambled eggs and substituted healthful granola cereal with raisins. His mid-morning snack was coffee and a "healthy" bran muffin, and lunch was a sandwich. Dinner was usually a pasta dish with generous helpings of whole-wheat bread. After a typical pasta dinner he'd feel dopey and tired. "I have a love-hate relationship with bread. I can't put it down, but it makes me feel stoned." There weren't more than a few grams of cholesterol in his diet, yet he couldn't keep his cholesterol down.

He seemed to be on a healthful diet—and he didn't even consume large amounts of refined sugar. What, then, was the problem? It had to do with something called the glycemic index.

A fascinating key to syndrome X—and to sugar disease in general—is the glycemic index. Until recently we viewed carbohydrates as either simple or complex sugars. When calculating the carbohydrate content of foods, we relied on the old "calorie bomb" concept, where foods were literally placed in a calorie furnace and burned. A baked potato might be equivalent in calories to a large bowl of brown rice, or three tablespoons of table sugar, because they all produced the same calorie burnoff. But their effects on the body are quite different, for our own energy-retrieval mechanisms are infinitely more complex and ultimately far more efficient than a furnace. Also, the effects vary remarkably from individual to individual. We now realize that there are factors that influence the speed with which carbohydrates are digested and sugar released into the body. As long ago as 1937, researchers found that the carbohydrate content of a food did not always correspond with the blood-sugar response it triggered. Dietary advice for anybody with a sugar problem *must* be based on this glycemic *response*—the actual change in blood sugar that occurs after a food is eaten.

Researchers at the University of Toronto and other centers have now established a glycemic index for foods, based on the blood-glucose level caused by the food in comparison with pure glucose.

The glycemic index is based on the concept that pure glucose has a 100 percent response—it is the ultimate, instantly usable sugar. High GIs create a characteristic high peak in a glucose-tolerance test, while low GIs create a kind of mild curve.

The results are shocking. Many foods we always thought were "good" carbohydrates may not be good for patients with sugar disease. Potatoes, for instance, have almost the same glycemic index as pure glucose. So do carrots and corn flakes. Whole wheat bread has a very high glycemic index, as do millet and white rice. Bananas and raisins, gram for gram, are as high as a Mars candy bar. Sucrose (refined sugar) has a lower index than brown rice or millet—and ice cream is even lower. Oddly enough, white flour in the form of spaghetti has a much lower glycemic index than white flour in the form of bread. The form of a food has a great impact on the way it changes blood-sugar levels: rice ground into flour has a much higher glycemic response.

Juices, most fruits, breads, and muffins (even the whole-grain, high-fiber kind) and even milk and yogurt (which contain milk sugar) have relatively high GIs. Surprising to some is the fact that dried fruit, despite its "naturalness," has a GI virtually identical with commercial candy.

The message is that not all that emanates from the health-food store is beneficial for patients with sugar disease. What's left? Legumes and *whole* grains in their unmilled form—like brown rice, barley, bulgur, rolled oats, teff (an Ethiopian grain), amaranth, and quinoa (South American grains). A cardinal rule: live as if the flour mill had never been invented. The milling process makes the starch inside grains more susceptible to digestion and rapid absorption of its sugar content. That is because flour products are more concentrated and the process of milling actually raises the glycemic index of a grain.

In addition, frequent small meals keep blood-sugar fluctuations to a minimum and conserve insulin. These guidelines are embodied in the Salad and Salmon Diet, which I have designed for patients with sugar disease. Carbohydrate-free foods such as meat, fish, poultry, salad, eggs, oils, and butter have GIs of zero.

GLYCEMIC INDEX OF SOME COMMON CARBOHYDRATE FOODS

Food Group	Percentage
Glucose (also known as dextrose)	100 percent
Corn flakes, carrots, parsnips, potatoes (instant mashed), maltose, honey	80–90 percent
Bread (white), millet, rice (white), potatoes	70–79 percent
Bread (whole meal), rice (brown), muesli, shredded wheat, bananas, raisins, Mars bar	60–69 percent
Buckwheat, spaghetti (white), sweet corn, peas, yams, sucrose (table sugar), potato chips	50–59 percent
Spaghetti (whole-wheat), oatmeal, sweet potatoes, beans, oranges, orange juice	40–49 percent
Butter beans, black-eyed peas, chick-peas, apples, ice cream, milk (skim and whole), plain yogurt	30–39 percent
Kidney beans, lentils	20–29 percent
Soybeans, peanuts	10–19 percent

No wonder my patient, with his family history of diabetes and heart disease, and his morning granola, raisins, apple juice, and evening

THE SALAD AND SALMON DIET

▼

A diet I frequently talk about on "Health Talk" and which I prescribe often for my patients is the Salad and Salmon Diet. This diet is extremely beneficial for weight loss, for cholesterol and blood-pressure reduction, and for diabetes control. It may also help minimize allergies in some patients. It is enjoyable and easy to follow and centers on delectable "spa cuisine."

Emphasize
Fish (especially fresh salmon, trout, tuna, and mackerel)
Shellfish, shrimp, lobster
Skinless breast of chicken or turkey
Tofu, beans, lentils, split peas, other legumes
Green leafy vegetables, salads, sprouts
Cabbage-family vegetables, tomatoes
One apple, pear, or orange or half a grapefruit per day
Eight glasses mineral or spring water per day
Four ounces whole grains per day (brown rice, millet, bulgur wheat, buckwheat, quinoa, amaranth, barley, rolled oats)
Two rice cakes per day
Olive, canola, or flaxseed oil
Sesame seeds, pumpkin seeds, sunflower seeds, walnuts, hazelnuts
Eight ounces plain low-fat yogurt
Garlic, cayenne, ginger, fresh spices
Olive oil and vinegar or lemon

Optional:
Eggs (poached or hard-boiled) three times a week

Avoid
Beef, veal, pork, lamb, organ meats, luncheon meats
Corn, potatoes, sweet potatoes, winter squash, carrots, beets
Other fruits, jams, jellies, fruit juice, dried fruit
Alcoholic beverages, sodas, vegetable juice
White rice and all flour products: breads, muffins, cookies, noodles, pasta, cakes, crackers, matzoh, breakfast cereals (except Wheatena, oatmeal, or oat bran)
Margarine, butter, lards, other oils
All other nuts, nut butters

(continued)

All other dairy products, frozen or flavored yogurt, Iced Bean, Rice Dream, or Tofutti
Salt, soy sauce
Ketchup, mayonnaise, commercial salad dressing
Breaded or fried foods, refined sugar, artificial sweeteners, honey, barley malt, maple syrup, rice syrup, and other natural sweeteners

pasta and bread, was suffering from syndrome X. His diet was "healthy," but it didn't take care of his blood-sugar problem.

Research on the glycemic index has provided some fascinating clues to diet and blood sugar. For instance, raw foods seem to be processed slower—and cause a flatter glycemic "curve" or response—than their cooked counterparts. Another amazing tidbit: the carbohydrate in one meal affects the digestion of the carbohydrate in the next meal. Slowly digested carbohydrates *improve* a person's carbohydrate tolerance of the next meal. A breakfast containing lentils (which have a very low glycemic index) will cause a flatter glycemic response to a standard lunch than a breakfast of bread. In fact, I often tell my patients to have split-pea or lentil soup for breakfast. It's an uncommon breakfast, but it starts the day off with a stable blood-sugar curve, thus reducing sugar cravings.

Another interesting fact? Foods eaten slowly and continuously in small, divided portions cause a much flatter glycemic index. Although it has a higher GI, bread eaten in small doses over four hours causes the same blood-sugar changes as lentils eaten in twenty minutes. (That may be one reason hypoglycemics are encouraged to eat frequent small meals.)

Some have proposed that people with variants of sugar disease follow a diet that rigidly excludes carbohydrates, concentrating instead on meat, oils, and leafy vegetables. In my opinion this is rarely necessary and results in dietary imbalance, inviting other degenerative conditions engendered by protein, cholesterol, and fat excess. Foods low in glycemic response should be emphasized.

Diabetes

It was not until 1674 that a brilliant anatomist and physician, Thomas Willis, first wrote about and named a new and extraordinary sweetness in the urine of his ill—and mostly wealthy—patients. He described this symptom of disease as diabetes (from the Greek word meaning inordinate passage of urine) mellitus (from the Latin word meaning honey). Around the time of his discovery, sugar consumption in England had soared to 16 million pounds a year.

Diabetes comes in two varieties: insulin-dependent (IDDM) and non–insulin-dependent (NIDDM). The former results from the body's failure to produce insulin; the latter usually from an overabundance of insulin. Both respond well to the measures I outline below for controlling sugar disease in general. But although patients with IDDM can reduce their insulin requirements, they can never do entirely without it.

Those with NIDDM, on the other hand, often require no medication if they follow a rigorous dietary and exercise program. One excellent example of that was an overweight patient who came to me with recently diagnosed diabetes, high triglycerides, and high cholesterol. Her physician, one of the top diabetes specialists in the city, recommended the diet prescribed by the American Diabetes Association. He also placed her on oral medication, which would stimulate the pancreas to produce more insulin. Unfortunately, this can ultimately worsen the cycle of insulin resistance and lead to full-blown diabetes requiring daily injections.

I explained to my patient that the 1,200-calorie diet recommended by the ADA was based on the old concept of calories and not on the state-of-the-art glycemic index. I asked her to get on the scale, and she refused, bursting into tears and explaining that her mother had always made a tremendous issue about the weight problem, so she did not want to weigh herself. I made a deal with her.

"Maria," I told her, "I'll never weigh you here. But this is a serious disease that threatens your life, and it has nothing to do with a mother trying to goad her reluctant daughter into losing weight. So the end point that I'll check with you on each visit is your blood sugar. As long as that's improving, your body weight is okay with me." I explained the glycemic index, put her on the Salad and Salmon Diet, and encouraged her to exercise and take nutritional supplements. I also recommended she check her blood sugar after every meal using a home finger-sticking kit, available in most drugstores. Often, non–insulin-dependent diabetics are told not to bother checking their blood sugar, since it's not essential to calculating the dose of their medicine. I find, however, that it is a profoundly important part of controlling any diabetes. A patient gains immediate and continuous feedback about blood-sugar levels, and about how different foods impact them. It's almost as if each meal becomes a mini-glucose-tolerance test, and the patient learns to correlate symptoms with actual blood-sugar levels.

The benefit to my patient was enormous. She is now off all medications. She also has lost weight (although she doesn't want to know how much)! And while she may not conform to her mother's ideal fashion-plate image, she's healthy, active, and at sixty-five contemplating opening her own word-processing business.

SWEET FACTS
▼

- We eat an average of 80 grams a day of sugar (excluding milk sugars).
- Of those 80 grams, about 53 are "added" sugar (not naturally present in foods).
- Two decades ago we used sucrose almost exclusively as an added sugar. Now we use sucrose, glucose, and fructose.
- When you feed your dog Gaines-burgers, Beef Bite Treats, Kibbles & Bits, or Butcher Bones, he is getting added sugar in the form of corn syrup, dextrose, or molasses. Your meat treat might be inducing syndrome X in your lethargic canine!

Excerpted from the *Report of Sugars Task Force*, published in *The Journal of Nutrition*, November 1986.

Determining Whether You Have Sugar Disease

As mentioned before, the glucose-tolerance test (GTT), even if performed for five consecutive hours, may sometimes provide the mistaken reassurance that a patient does not suffer from sugar disease. Even patients who feel devastated by the sugar challenge used in the GTT are often told not to worry, that they have no problem, that their symptoms have no *real* basis. The answer lies in designing a better, more sensitive GTT.

How is this accomplished? At my office, we not only measure blood sugar at each of several designated times, we also measure the body's insulin response, as well as the production of adrenaline at the crucial instant where blood sugar "bottoms out" and symptoms occur. This assures that even when glucose levels are normal, any abnormality in metabolism will be appreciated. A hypoglycemia index can be calculated also, by applying a mathematical formula to the glucose results obtained. The index takes into account not just how low blood sugar dips but also how rapidly it occurs. The result: more accurate testing for hypoglycemia, syndrome X, and unsuspected diabetic tendency.

If you are interested in measuring your body's insulin response, and your hypoglycemia index, suggest it to your doctor.

Good Fats

While all fats get a bad rap because of their high calorie content, in the treatment of sugar disease there are "good guy" fats and "bad guy" fats. Saturated fats, such as those found in modern feedlot-raised livestock, seem to hasten the development of sugar disease. In addition, altered fats like margarine and hydrogenated oils may impair the body's carbohydrate metabolism while adding unwanted pounds.

Conversely, Omega-3 oils—such as those found in flax seed and coldwater fish like salmon, trout, and tuna, or the wild game our ancestors ate—help curb insulin resistance. Monounsaturated fats—found in olive oil and canola—also help adjust blood sugar.

Supplements

A key supplement for treating sugar disease is chromium. A question I'm frequently asked is: "If chromium is helpful in diabetes, how can it be helpful for the opposite condition—hypoglycemia?" The answer lies in the unique ability of chromium to enhance the action of insulin—allowing the body to step down its production of the critical hormone. This results in fewer highs and lows.

A variety of herbs help maintain blood sugar, and even attenuate sugar craving: Gymnema Sylvestre, the ancient Ayurvedic "sugar destroyer"; stevia, an Amazonian herb, a noncaloric sweet sugar equivalent; and fenugreek, a mild, natural blood-sugar lowerer. Garlic, too, helps lower blood sugar, and has a lipid-regulating effect.

It's not uncommon for many of my diabetic patients to reduce or eliminate their medication. We put them on the Salad and Salmon Diet (see page 82). The diet emphasizes low glycemic-index foods, weighted toward Omega-3 and monounsaturated fats.

Exercise

Exercise is a great "leveler" for persons with sugar disease. Studies show that mild, regular aerobic exercise of short duration—like power walking twenty minutes a day—can forestall the development of diabetes in susceptible individuals, or reverse it when it has already occurred. I've found aerobic exercise helpful, too, for hypoglycemics—it helps to stabilize troublesome autonomic nervous system symptoms and makes patients more resilient. Exercise is certainly an antidote to mid-abdominal weight gain that is a hallmark of syndrome X.

Smoking

Smokers may sometimes have hidden sugar disease. They often pick up a cigarette instead of sweets, not because there is sugar in tobacco smoke but because the nicotine in tobacco has a powerful effect on the entire body. In particular, nicotine causes glucose that is stored in the liver to be released into the bloodstream. This may be one reason that some people who quit smoking eat more than before—they simply can't handle the food cravings and weight gain. Efforts should be made *before* quitting to address an individual's sugar craving and possible hypoglycemia by adopting a proper diet, rich in foods that have a low glycemic index. According to studies, although smoking helps some people keep thin, even lean smokers have higher waist/hip ratios than their nonsmoking counterparts. And quitting smoking, according to the latest findings, reduces insulin resistance.

One question you may have after reading so much about the dangers of sugar is: Why do we crave a substance so seemingly harmful? Did nature go awry?

Not really. There was once a profound survival mechanism in our sweet tooth, for in the plant kingdom, many of the foods with a sugary taste are also the most beneficial and nutritious—from fruits to squash and carrots. (In contrast, many poisonous foods contain toxic alkaloids

DO YOU HAVE SUGAR DISEASE?

▼

1. Do you have an elevated waist-to-hip ratio? Get a tape measure and measure your waist/hip ratio. If it's greater than 1.0 for males or 0.8 for women, you may have a problem. Feel for your hipbones on the side to locate the hip, measure them, then measure your waist and calculate. For instance, if you are a male, and your waist is 36 and your hips are 34, your ratio is greater than 1, and you may be in trouble.

2. Do you have a love-hate relationship with pasta and breads? Do you crave them but find that after eating them you feel tired?

3. When you're depressed, do you eat sweets?

4. During the winter months, do you eat more sweets? (Studies show that some people suffer from a form of depression, seasonal affective disorder, that only occurs during the winter months when they aren't exposed to much sunlight. A concomitant of SAD is sugar craving.)

5. Do you sometimes get weak, irritable, and shaky and find that these symptoms are relieved by eating sugar?

6. Do you wake in the middle of the night feeling hungry?

Score one point for each yes answer. Rate yourself as follows:
0 points: you're fine.
1–2 points: mild sugar disease
3–4 points: moderate sugar disease
5–6 points: serious sugar disease

that have a bitter taste, and it was a general rule of thumb that sweet was nutritious and bitter was toxic.) We had a tremendous drive to seek out these foods, but they were seasonal and, in spite of their sweet taste, not nearly as abundant in sugar as a typical modern dessert, like apple pie à la mode. Finding pure sugar was an extremely arduous process: Indians, for instance, spent long hours tapping sap-laden trees in late winter, and laboriously cooking the syrup in wooden bins to distill and purify it. This was hardly akin to driving to the supermarket and picking up a six-pack of sweet soft drinks.

Sugar can affect mood profoundly. Sugar consumption can, over many years, cause constant, stressful insulin surges that seriously damage your health. If you can cut refined sugars from your diet, you may find yourself both more energized and calmer. This simple change could alter your life.

Your Energy Plan

Take the quiz in this chapter. If you think you may be suffering from low blood sugar, ask your doctor for an oral glucose-tolerance test. If you have symptoms during the test—even if he tells you it is normal—consider the possibility that you have sugar disease. You can also ask your doctor to measure your insulin and adrenaline during this test. A hypoglycemia index can be calculated to see how rapidly blood sugar dips.

Your treatment:

• Cut off your intake of sugar.
• Switch to the Salad and Salmon Diet, a diet that emphasizes foods with a *low* glycemic index.
• Avoid flour and bread, which cause the blood sugar to peak faster than whole grains.
• Eat good-guy fats like Omega-3 oils found in cold-water fish. Also emphasize monounsaturated fats like olive and canola oil. They help even out blood sugar.
• Take chromium, a supplement that enhances the action of insulin, allowing the body to step down its production of this critical hormone.

Tired All the Time

• Reduce sugar craving with herbs such as Gymnema Sylvestre, stevia, and fenugreek.

• Exercise. Studies show that mild, regular aerobic exercise will reverse diabetes or hypoglycemia.

• Stop smoking.

• Don't "sneak" sugar in the form of barley malt, rice syrup, or other so-called "natural" sugars.

• If you have full-blown diabetes, use the finger-sticking home test after every meal. This will give you immediate feedback about foods and your blood-sugar levels and help you adjust your diet.

6

PLAYING DIET DETECTIVE: ARE THE FOODS YOU CHOOSE MAKING YOU TIRED?

▼

As we've seen, the endocrine system constitutes an important part of your fatigue wheel. When your hormones are in balance, you are not subject to the exhausting swings of premenstrual syndrome, sugar blues, or adrenal exhaustion. But hormones are only one piece of the pie.

Another huge—and often overlooked—source of fatigue is food. The very substances that are supposed to nourish us can sometimes cause chronic fatigue. Playing diet detective can make a major difference in your energy levels. Often my patients are astonished at the way eliminating a few simple foods can "magically" banish exhaustion.

One of my lab technicians used to come to our Thursday morning rounds—where I gather my staff to discuss new procedures, difficult cases, and laboratory protocol—and plunk himself in a comfortable chair. Within minutes he would be snoring. Many times I took him aside afterward to ask why he wasn't getting enough sleep and, in particular, why he was burning the candle at both ends the night before rounds. His inevitable and heartfelt protestation was, "Dr. Hoffman, I get plenty of sleep, but I'm tired every morning. I don't know why."

I queried him about his breakfast, and he confessed to a passion for corn muffins. We tested him for allergy to a variety of foods and found that corn provoked itching, yawning, and sleepiness. He eliminated his morning muffins; after that, he was alert at rounds.

You have probably heard and read a lot about food allergy, and you may have encountered widely divergent and contradictory views. It is a field beset with controversy. On the one hand are conventional allergists who view food allergy as an extremely rare and violent response—the kind of life-threatening reaction that causes a person to break out in hives or go into anaphylactic shock. (In anaphylactic shock, blood pressure plummets and the throat and bronchial tubes close.) For those individuals who are truly and perilously allergic to a food, even a single nut or bite of shrimp can be potentially fatal. Most allergists believe that only severe symptoms like sudden diarrhea, vomiting, hives, swelling, or shock are indications of true food allergies.

Classical food allergies ignite a component of the immune system called IgE—and they produce an immediate, direct response. The immune system mistakes a harmless substance, such as milk or corn, for an invader from the outside—such as a bacteria or virus. This sets off a chain reaction of attack, with the production of a cascade of IgE antibodies. They grab hold of the invaders and set off another chain reaction that concludes with the release of potent chemicals, like histamine. These chemicals cause uncomfortable and even devastating symptoms.

For many of us, the response is more diffuse, can occur hours later, and may be regulated by other components of the immune system. I myself am an allergy "zealot"—I believe that allergies are profuse and widespread in our society and that they can even occasionally be a contributor to mental illness, attention-deficit disorder in children, and countless chronic conditions.

I contend that in countless people certain foods produce a mild and constant stress that can indeed be a source of chronic problems, most often fatigue. In strict terms, this is a food intolerance rather than a true allergy. (Through most of this chapter I will nevertheless refer to food reactions as "allergies." They are not classic allergies, but the word is convenient and easy to understand.) These intolerances can stress the body in subtle ways each day, leading to a constant state of low energy. An easy way to test for these intolerances is simply to fast for one to four days and see if your energy level rises dramatically.

Food allergy is a complex web—reactions to food are modulated by how much is consumed, how often it is eaten, and whether or not other allergens or toxins are stressing the body. In some cases, it's quite possible the immune system is directly involved. For instance,

IS FOOD ALLERGY REAL?

▼

There are many studies on food allergy, some of which seem to prove it doesn't exist while others maintain the opposite. Research by S. Allan Bock, an allergist at the National Jewish Center for Immunology and Respiratory Medicine in Denver, found that 65 percent of nearly 500 children diagnosed with food allergies showed no symptoms when tested in a double-blind study. (Neither the child nor the physician knew whether he was giving the child a capsule containing a suspect food or a placebo. This is called a traditional double-blind study, which is the gold standard of scientific research. Both subject and physician are unaware of what the patient is actually getting, so that the placebo effect is eliminated and results are objective.) But critics question whether food challenge with capsules is the same as eating a food.

Other research has shown the opposite. One well-designed study of 88 English children suffering from migraines and other symptoms found that 78 recovered completely and were symptom-free after being placed on diets free of possible allergenic foods; 40 of the children were then tested in a double-blind follow-up study, and 35 became ill after consuming the allergenic foods.

many foods contain lectins. These short-chain molecules interact with proteins, causing them to coagulate in the patterns used by hospital labs to detect blood types. Since certain lectins react only with certain blood types, it is possible that certain foods trigger reactions only in genetically susceptible individuals. This theory was proposed by Peter D'Adamo, the son of a Connecticut naturopath. He claims to have worked out a system matching blood types to food sensitivities. It is an interesting notion but is a long way from acceptance by most doctors.

One has only to see the astonishing results of a simple elimination diet in many patients to become a believer in the power of food allergy. Patients come to my office complaining of chronic fatigue, muscle aches, depression, *and* cravings for foods, and as soon as they eliminate common allergy-causing foods from their diet, they feel renewed, even exhilarated.

Another tipoff to food allergies is daily craving for a particular food. As you may recall from Chapter 2, when the body adapts to an allergen it may actually become habituated to the presence of that substance. It is not uncommon for patients with food allergies unwittingly to eat the same food in different forms every day: cereal with milk in the morning, a grilled cheese sandwich for lunch, and pizza or vegetables au gratin for dinner. The common elements—in this case, wheat and dairy—may indeed be allergens.

An estimated 30 million Americans experience adverse reactions to foods. How is it that we've come to be so sensitive to food, our sustenance and lifeline?

Think of the foods that fill our supermarket shelves and restaurants. What looks like a cornucopia of varied comestibles is deceptive. Our common, ubiquitous foods happen to be the leading causes of food intolerance: dairy products, eggs, nuts, soybeans, wheat, corn. Even when we don't think we're eating these foods, we may be consuming them unwittingly in some form. Corn appears in many foods in the form of corn syrup and cornstarch. Casein, a milk protein, is used in breads, sauces, and baked goods.

A primitive hunter-gatherer diet was far different. It consisted mostly of succulent roots and shoots, berries, leafy foliage, and wild game, and food rotated with the seasons. Our bodies, in the brief moment of eternity that has passed since we evolved out of the wild, may not have adapted yet to these monotonous foods of civilization.

Take the case of gluten, the protein part of certain grains, such as barley, rye, oats, and wheat. Gluten is a relatively novel food in the human food chain, and in many cultures it did not exist until recently. Gluten intolerance in certain individuals is responsible for a severe systemic disorder known as celiac disease, a severe intestinal inflammation that causes constant diarrhea and weight loss. It is also well known that relatives of people who suffer from celiac disease often have a low-grade manifestation of this ailment. In these individuals, the villi, the microscopic fingerlike projections on the intestinal wall that are crucial to proper food absorption, become flattened and damaged. There may be no obvious and dramatic disease, but these individuals may not absorb their nutrients efficiently, and they may have low-grade symptoms of bloating and fatigue.

Another possible cause of food allergy is what some doctors like to call the leaky-gut syndrome (see Chapter 7). In some individuals, chronic intestinal inflammation is created by an imbalance of bacteria, yeast, or parasites. The unhealthy microbes proliferate, and they tend to produce harmful toxins that can inflame the intestine. This inflamed intestine forms an imperfect barrier through which undigested food particles may pass straight into the bloodstream, where they are perceived by the body as foreign invaders. Clearing up bowel inflammation, and restoring a healthy balance of good bacteria, can often clear up food allergies.

Perhaps the most frustrating aspect of food allergy is the fact that many people are allergic to their favorite foods—the ones they eat every day. The thought of giving up those beloved foods is pure anguish. But the good news is that, in most cases, if you eliminate an allergenic food for several months, you will be able to tolerate it again—as long as you eat it only once or twice a week. The key is moderation.

There are several ways your doctor can test for food allergy. One is a blood test called the RAST, which measures the levels of IgE or IgG (both immunoglobulins that form antibodies to foods) in your blood. Another is a skin test, where an extract of the food is scratched or injected under your skin to see if you develop an allergic welt that looks like a mosquito bite.

These tests are helpful, but they do not tell the whole story of food allergy. Food reactions are very hard to pin down, and they may occur instantly or they may show up several hours after you've eaten a food. They can trigger a whole range of symptoms, and they can wax and wane. For instance, food allergies may worsen during great stress or during the hay-fever season.

The one surefire way to find out whether you're allergic to a food is to eliminate it. Then, after four days have passed, eat it again. Your body will have deadapted (see Chapter 2), and your symptoms will reappear in a marked and obvious manner when you eat the food again. You'll know you're allergic.

The elimination diet is so effective that it is important for your doctor to oversee it. You need to be carefully monitored, and in many cases the allergenic foods need to be reintroduced in very tiny doses, as small as half a teaspoon, to protect you from a highly unpleasant and violent reaction.

Most individuals are allergic to more than one food. I've developed

DO YOU HAVE HIDDEN FOOD ALLERGIES?

▼

Suspect hidden food allergies if you suffer from some of the following symptoms:

- fatigue
- dark circles under your eyes
- anxiety, irritability, depression, fogginess
- chronic sinus infection, coughing, or wheezing
- digestive problems
- frequent headaches, muscle aches, or joint pains
- itching and skin problems
- chronic sore throat

Ask yourself the following seven questions:

1. Do you crave certain foods?

2. Do you feel different on weekends? Food patterns often shift from the week to the weekends. For instance, people who drink coffee at work may skip it on weekends and suffer caffeine-withdrawal headaches. Similarly, when people travel and eat a different cuisine, their allergy symptoms may wax or wane.

3. Do you have food fixations? Do you eat a single type of food in different forms during the day (muffins for breakfast, a sandwich for lunch, and pasta for dinner)?

4. Do you have energy cycles? Do you alternate between states of tension and irritability and states of sleepy exhaustion?

5. Do you feel better when you don't eat anything at all?

6. Do you have a family history of allergies? Do your relatives suffer from hay fever, eczema, or asthma?

7. Does your pulse become more rapid after eating a particular food? Sit down and relax, and take your pulse at the wrist. A normal reading is 52–70 beats per minute. Now eat the suspected food, wait fifteen minutes, and take your pulse again. If it has increased more than ten beats per minute, try omitting this food from your diet.

Playing Diet Detective

a three-stage elimination diet that gradually tests groups of food. I also sometimes use an oligoantigenic diet, which means a diet without any likely allergens (or food antigens). There are oligoantigenic protein powders available. One, called Vivonex, is available by prescription. Another, called UltraClear, is available through nutritionists and doctors but is not a prescription powder. Both are complete and nutritionally balanced meal-replacement beverages, carefully formulated so that even the most sensitive individuals are able to utilize them. They contain predigested proteins that the body can assimiliate instantly. These beverages give allergic individuals a rest and allow the body time to wash out its toxic load of allergens and immune complexes.

One unconventional way to treat food allergies is to give a patient allergy shots—just as traditional allergists desensitize a hay-fever sufferer to pollens. This controversial approach can sometimes work beautifully. The introduction of minute amounts of suspected foods—either via shots or under the tongue—can gradually condition the body to accept such foods.

A vivid example is how my lab director cured his wife of a severe

SULFITE ALLERGIES

▼

Food allergies are sometimes due to the effect of chemicals in processed foods. Colorings, additives, residues of hormones and pesticides, and other traces of chemicals may cause some people to react profoundly. They may walk around thinking they have a hundred different food allergies when in truth they are reacting to one or two chemical substances that are added to many foods.

For instance, some people are extremely sensitive to sulfites. There is now a product called Sulfitest, which contains test strips that detect the presence of sulfites in foods. Write for information to: Center Laboratories, Division of EM Industries, Port Washington, New York 11050. Sulfites are commonly added to the following foods and beverages: avocado dip, beer, carrots, cider, coleslaw, frozen doughs, frozen fruits and vegetables, fruits, gelatin, lettuce, mushrooms, peppers, pickles, potatoes, shellfish, shrimp, tomatoes, and many wines.

shrimp allergy. She's a Filipino, and shrimp is a major food in her cuisine. Yet her reactions to shrimp were almost life-threatening. Taking a cue from modern allergy theory, and unbeknownst to me, he started introducing extraordinarily small quantities of shrimp into her diet. She ate these tiny amounts without ill effect, moved on to larger doses, and eventually built a tolerance. Now she can eat shrimp without a reaction. (Don't try this unorthodox approach on your own, unless it is under a professional allergist's supervision. You might end up in the hospital.)

Just as ingenious was the way a beekeeper I met years ago received a cure to his allergy to bee stings. He told me that one day in the 1950s a hive toppled over him and he was stung by at least 300 bees. The insult was such a profound one that thereafter every time a single bee stung him he had a major allergic reaction. Beekeeping was his life's work, and he didn't want to relinquish it. Instead he went to an innovative New York City allergist who asked him to collect a few of his bees and *bring them into the office!* She prepared a special extract of their venom and instructed him to give himself progressively higher doses until he could tolerate bee stings again. It worked!

The beekeeper's experience illustrates a principle of allergy that applies to food as well. A sporadic exposure to a substance can usually be tolerated by the immune system. But constant or extraordinary exposure (such as wheat or milk five or six times a day) can overwhelm the immune response. Remember that our ancestors ate only seasonal food and that they hunted and foraged in times of both feast and famine. When there was famine, they were forced to undergo a natural "fast," which may have allowed their bodies to detoxify and rebalance.

Although allergy is an important aspect of food intolerance, I don't look at food and fatigue only in terms of allergy, which is a small part of the story where the impact of food on energy is concerned. There are some new studies in the forefront of research in the area of food that provide some fascinating clues to how foods may work like drugs in our bodies—and strongly affect our moods and energy levels. And an intriguing new theory suggests that we may actually fall into specific metabolic "types"—each type suited to different categories of food. Some of us may benefit from raw foods, some from vegetarian diets, others from heavy doses of meat. The reason may be simple enough:

our ancestral roots are diverse, and some of our ancestors may have carved their evolutionary niche on the sparse savannah; others may have inhabited lush rain forests, and still others may have braved the near-arctic conditions of the far north. Each part of the world has different patterns of food consumption, and so some of us may be carrying the hereditary imprint of meat-eating tundra dwellers, while others have inherited a digestive system built to handle lots of tropical fruit and fresh vegetables. That may be why some of us are virtually cholesterol-proof no matter how high-fat our diets. Similarly, descendants of Native Americans often succumb to the devastating effects of high-calorie, high-fat American foods by developing diabetes, while the descendants of Scandinavian immigrants can eat meat with relative impunity and adapt better—although not always perfectly—to the standard American diet.

One profound way that foods can cause allergy and fatigue is by affecting the microbe balance in the gut. A leading British researcher, J. O. Hunter, recently proposed an interesting new theory in the prestigious British medical journal *The Lancet*. He believes that the gut is not just a tube but a complex chemical factory in which foods are broken down in different ways. These ways are dependent on the specific bacterial or fungal balance in the intestines. Certain microbes may literally ferment sugar into alcohol, while others may break it down into toxic aldehydes. Both processes can create profound fatigue, since alcohol and aldehydes stress the whole system, particularly the liver. Still other microbes may yield unusual chemicals that may act as neurotransmitters in the brain. This process may vary from individual to individual—for each person has a different genetic inheritance and carries around his own unique balance of gut bacteria. One person may literally get drunk from fruit juice, while another can drink it with no such effect. One individual may get a lift from eating meat, while another may feel drowsy as a lion after devouring its prey. Dr. Hunter calls these "entero-metabolic food reactions," and it certainly helps explain how foods can tire some of us out while others can eat the same foods and remain energetic.

Another fascinating new theory is one promulgated by Jonathan Brostoff, a leading British physician who has marshaled intriguing evidence to show that foods can act as if they were drugs in several powerful ways. Brostoff contends that enzyme defects—the inability

Tired All the Time

of the body to inactivate or detoxify certain substances because of a lack of certain natural chemical catalysts—are far more common than we realize. Seventy percent of the adult population in the world has trouble digesting milk. Of the world population, North Americans and Europeans are best able to tolerate milk, and even so, many of us have dairy allergies.

Although lactose (milk protein) intolerance is not a strict allergy, it can cause bloating, gas, and fatigue. Brostoff believes people may become allergic or sensitive to foods because their enzyme systems have been battered—either because they inherited faulty systems or because the environment has stressed and weakened them. One study of 80 food-sensitive patients found that they were slow metabolizers of certain chemicals—and had problems not only with foods but also with detoxifying certain drugs. Their bodies were slower at this detoxification process than were those of healthy individuals.

How does this translate to foods? One fascinating example occurs in the case of phenol compounds. Phenols are contained in almost all foods—and in particularly high levels in milk, coffee, and fruits. They are considered "insoluble" acids, and need to be detoxified and excreted by liver enzymes. Phenols may be the cause of food intolerance in certain individuals who cannot inactivate and dispose of these chemicals as quickly as others. Alcohol is known to inhibit the necessary enzymes, and that may be one reason that alcohol plus a meal high in phenols may bring on a migraine or a sensitivity reaction. That reaction stresses the body and inevitably causes fatigue.

Another, remarkably overlooked mechanism by which food causes fatigue is by acting exactly like a drug. Our body produces its own internal morphinelike chemicals, endogenous opiates (called endorphins). These feel-good chemicals help reduce pain and produce euphoria. Is it just a coincidence that wheat and milk have chains of amino acids that are remarkably similar to our internal morphine? Not only does a plate of pastry or a bowl of ice cream calm us down—it may even make us sleepy. Perhaps when some patients stop eating grains and dairy, their increased energy is due to the fact that their bodies aren't doped by the opiatelike chemicals in certain foods.

Evidence seems to suggest this may be true. Patients suffering from bulimia often binge on just such foods, and one reason may be that they are abnormally sensitive to exactly those chemicals in foods. When certain patients were given a morphine antagonist—a drug that blocks the effect of endorphins—they recovered from their bulimia. One possible therapy for severely food-addicted and food-fatigued patients might be to give them such a drug temporarily.

Another point that Brostoff makes is that allergy, even when it's "in the mind," is legitimately in the body. Allergy can simply be a conditioned response. People may be allergic to certain foods, have adverse reactions, and begin to experience eating as a perilous venture. The situation is not unlike that of someone who has experienced panic attacks in public and is now afraid to leave the house. And the response isn't limited to human beings. Even guinea pigs, in experiments, can be conditioned to become "allergic" to harmless substances. This can happen if the harmless substance is given along with an allergen, so that the guinea pigs associate the two substances. Soon they will react to either one.

Finally, allergy may be due to a genuine deficiency in the immune system. If this deficiency is not too severe, one can eliminate allergenic foods, but it is also important to help boost the immune system through good nutrition, supplements, and rest. The most allergic woman I've ever seen was a patient who had had mild asthma in childhood and in her twenties went to a doctor complaining of slight hair loss. Her physician was chief of endocrinology at a major university hospital, and I've never understood why, but he prescribed steroids for her symptoms. This aggressive steroid therapy went on for years, until she became dependent. She finally went to another doctor, who explained the dangers of steroids and weaned her off them (she also successfully sued the first doctor for malpractice), but by that time her immune system was crippled. Once she was off steroids she developed severe eczema all over her body, and reported that she was allergic to every single food she ate. Peanuts and fish actually caused her throat to close, but all foods made her itch.

I was skeptical, but when I tested her with a RAST, her total level of IgE was so high it was unmeasurable. It was beyond the detection limits of the test. In addition, she was allergic to every single food on the test. I also discovered that she had a deficiency in some crucial immune globulins, the body's natural defense substances. Because the test results justified the treatment, I prescribed gamma globulin infusions. These cost up to $1,200 per infusion (because the purification process is delicate and labor-intensive) and had to be given every three weeks. Her condition was so extreme that her insurance company covered the cost. Using this sophisticated technology, we can help reconstitute her immune system, but she may be dependent on these infusions for life. Another useful immune booster is called transfer factor—a mixture of crucial immune substances purified from the blood of healthy donors. It is hard to obtain and has been used only in the most intractable and severe allergy cases.

Still another hopeful strategy for dealing with intractable food allergies is enzyme-potentiated desensitization (EPD), developed by British physician Len McEwen. EPD involves periodic skin vaccinations with food mixtures that have had their efficacy "boosted" by the addition of specific immune-potentiating enzymes. The therapy is currently offered by only a handful of physicians in the United States and Great Britain as an investigational treatment.

Patients who suspect they have food allergies may wonder if it is worth all the trouble avoiding foods they love. Elimination diets can sound bewildering and rigorous. Some individuals would just prefer to be tired, in particular because some of us have a genetic susceptibility to certain allergies, and even if we try to clean up the gut, we may develop the same imbalances when we return to a "normal" diet. How can we follow a strict diet in a world that presents us with thousands of opportunities to eat the very foods that may be unhealthful for us?

I'm not saying it is easy to eliminate suspect foods, but selective eating is so important for lifelong health that I think it is worth it. We are adrift in an eating environment that is highly unnatural. We need to devote more time to thinking about food and its effects on our body. If society is ready to unleash powerful drugs to treat everything from ulcers to cancer, why do we take such a blasé approach to our diet? Let us not talk just about aggressive management of medical conditions. Let us talk about aggressive prevention, through healthful diets, keyed to our specific nutritional needs and attuned to our intolerances.

So many people can combat their fatigue through a healthy diet that it seems worthwhile to check your own diet for hidden food allergies. Even if you're thinking, "This sounds complicated," I can promise you it's worth it.

Playing Diet Detective

Your Energy Plan

The cheapest and most efficient way to test for food allergies is to eliminate suspect foods. See my previous book *Seven Weeks to a Settled Stomach* for a detailed description. It takes only three weeks, and it may eliminate years of malaise and fatigue, restoring you to health and energy.

For confirmation of food allergies, ask for a RAST test, which includes total levels of IgE.

To test a specific food allergy, cut out a food for four days, then eat it and take your pulse. If it speeds up more than 10 beats a minute, the food is probably suspect.

Rotate your foods, instead of eating the same food in different forms three times a day. In other words, if you have wheat for breakfast, don't also eat wheat in a slice of pizza at lunch and in pasta at dinner. (Eat these every fourth day.)

Seek out a physician or allergist who is willing to neutralize you to allergenic foods. Contact the American Academy of Environmental Medicine, P.O. Box 16106, Denver, Colorado 80216 (303-622-9755), for a listing of such doctors.

See Chapter 7 on detoxification of the gut, which can help eliminate food allergies.

Try cutting out wheat, which is a common allergenic food and contains opiatelike substances that may make you feel sleepy and lethargic.

In extremely severe cases, where allergies to numerous foods exist and blood tests suggest immune deficiencies, consider boosting the immune system with transfer factor, immune globulins, or EPD.

7

THE INNER ENVIRONMENT: TOXINS WITHIN

▼

Let's say you've targeted your allergenic foods and eliminated them and you still feel fatigued. If you suffer from chronic fatigue, and especially if you suffer from the symptoms of food allergy and irritable bowel syndrome (gas, bloating, diarrhea, nausea, and discomfort), you may need to do more than simply clean up your diet. You may actually need to cleanse your internal piping.

You see, food allergies don't usually pop up out of nowhere. Usually they are linked to toxicity of the gut, which leads to an inflamed gut lining that allows undigested food particles to "leak" through into the blood, causing allergic reactions and chronic tiredness.

Internal cleansing can help restore and heal an inflamed gut. It's a method as old as man. Primitive tribesmen used to eat chunks of wet clay, according to anthropologists. The strange ritual called *geophagy,* or clay eating, was one way that primitive peoples had of detoxifying themselves. Even modern primates seem genetically programmed to seek and eat clay. (That may be one basis of pica, the tendency to eat dust and dirt that gets inner-city kids into trouble when they consume lead paint chips.) Clays are known for their adsorbstive capacity—that's why "mud packs" are a popular feature of facial treatments. Mud can pull harmful toxins out of the body.

Primitive man understood that toxins are not just invaders from the outside. So did the Greeks and Romans, who prescribed fasting and purging regimens. Your own body can be a breeding ground for harmful microbes and chemicals. Even animals seem to instinctively sense this: chimps in Tanzania, for instance, sometimes get up in the early morning, skip their usual breakfast of fruit, and walk fifteen or twenty minutes in search of Aspilia, a member of the sunflower family.

Tired All the Time

They gulp the leaves whole and then wrinkle their noses or even vomit. Clearly, the stuff tastes bad, but the leaves contain a red oil called thiarubrine-A that kills parasites, fungi, and viruses.

One of the primary sites of toxins in the body is the colon. Three trillion bacteria live in your gut. Many of these bacteria are beneficial, and help produce important vitamins (like vitamin K) as well as limit the growth of other, harmful microbes. The colon becomes toxic when those harmful bacteria, fungi, and parasites proliferate. These microbes feed on undigested food, producing toxic waste products such as ammonia. These products may irritate the lining of the gut, but studies have also shown that the presence of such bacteria can actually trigger an inflammatory immune reaction, causing remote reactions in other parts of the body. Sometimes these bacteria can even help initiate an autoimmune disease to which a person is already genetically predisposed. One such disease is known as ankylosing spondylitis, a painful lower-back problem in which the spine and pelvis become gradually fused. The ailment is thought by some to be triggered by the body's response to certain intestinal bacteria.

Intestinal flora—particularly yeasts—can even ferment sugars into alcohol. Ethyl alcohol was found in the blood of 311 out of 510 volunteers an hour after ingestion of 5 grams of glucose. Before the test, the volunteers had fasted for three hours, and they had had no alcohol at all for twenty-four hours. Gut microbes have been shown to ferment so much sugar into alcohol that blood levels were nearly 20 mg/100 ml of blood—exactly the level that constitutes drunk driving in Sweden!

How does the gut become toxic? It's pretty easy. First, start by being bottle-fed as a baby. Breast milk contains colostrum, which contains immune factors and antibodies. These go straight into the gut of a child—which initially is not fully developed—and prime it to have its own natural immune system. You may be surprised to learn that the gut has an immune system, but in fact there is an immunological barrier all along the lining of the gut that protects it.

Cow's milk, in contrast, may be sensitizing to the baby. The milk protein in cow's milk often creates allergies. Many babies with colic are actually experiencing an allergy to cow's milk. A baby fed cow's milk may start life with an inflamed gut wall.

To bottle feeding, add chlorinated and fluoridated tap water. Both kill bacteria, the good kinds as well as the bad. Chlorine may make your drinking water "safe" but it can also disrupt the growth and development of normal bacteria in the bowel.

Then, at the first sign of a cold, sore throat, or ear infection, add a course of antibiotics. Repeat that again and again. Add some more antibiotics to your diet with meat and milk from animals that have been dosed with antibiotics and hormones. Livestock ingest over 12 million pounds of antibiotics a year—more than humans consume. And sometimes they are dosed with "illegal" antibiotics—ones that are potentially harmful to humans but have escaped the vigilance of the FDA in regard to animals.

Antibiotics are notorious "weed" killers that poison not only the bad guys but also the good-guy bacteria that form a protective coating on the gut wall. As a result, simple fungi such as yeast and bacteria such as staph can proliferate, upsetting the balance of flora. Scientists noticed this over forty years ago: antibiotics, they found, not only caused a rapid increase in fungal illnesses, they seemed to intensify the virulence of candida as well. Antibiotics stimulate candida to convert from its regular yeast form to an invasive fungal form. In the fungal form, candida actually sends roots into the gut wall.

A hospital visit or two can also add to colon toxicity. Hospitals breed super germs—germs with names that most people can't even pronounce—because seriously ill people often fall victim to powerful strains of mutant bacteria and fungi that need huge doses of antibiotics to kill them. These mutant strains spread through the hospital and can colonize other patients. Studies of hospital workers show that their skin and feces are colonized with pathogenic bacteria. Most hospital workers don't get sick because their immune systems keep these unusual microbes at bay, but they lie in wait, dormant, until the time is ripe. Their presence in the GI tract may trigger subtle, undetected systemic reactions.

Other factors contribute as well. Certain fungi and yeast are stimulated by hormones, and so a woman taking birth-control pills is more susceptible to the growth of these microbes. Or a person who drinks a great deal of alcohol may partially sterilize his own gut, upsetting the balance further. Add aspirin, acetaminophen, or ibuprofen every time you get a fever, and you deprive your body of one of nature's best antibiotics. Bacteria live best at about 97 degrees. A fever helps weaken the bacteria and allows the immune system to gain the upper hand.

Eating lots of refined, high-sugar foods instead of fresh, enzyme-rich fruits and vegetables further poisons the colon. Antibiotic-laden meat is another problem—one study in the *American Journal of Public Health* found that individuals who consume antibiotic-treated poultry are more than twice as likely to come down with gastroenteritis than those who do not. In addition, toxins like excess alcohol in the diet can lead to reduced stomach acid and impaired digestive enzymes. A diet high in refined foods also slows the transit time in the colon, allowing toxins to linger and inflame the gut lining. Malabsorption, or leaky-gut syndrome, results.

What ends up happening to this abnormal intestinal milieu? The gut responds to the pathogenic bacteria by sending signals to the immune system that an unwelcome visitor is present. The immune system may then flail out, particularly in genetically susceptible individuals, causing symptoms eerily similar to the flu: achiness, fatigue, malaise. Often the inflammatory reaction inadvertently damages a part of the body—the joints in rheumatoid arthritis, the muscles in myositis, the gut itself in inflammatory bowel disease.

For a long time, the typical patient with leaky-gut syndrome was one eating a Western diet high in animal fats and bereft of fiber. The importance of fiber gained international attention when Colin Burkitt, a British physician, traveled the world and discovered that the incidence of many digestive diseases was much lower in parts of the third world where diets were high in fiber.

However, today I'm seeing a new breed of patients with digestive problems. They're more sophisticated about diet, and they limit saturated fats while emphasizing fiber. Nonetheless, many of them have chronic digestive problems for just the opposite reason: constant ingestion of hard-to-digest carbohydrates. The cure for digestive ills is not simply fiber, just as the "cure" for heart disease is not simply to lower cholesterol.

Many more people than you would think suffer from carbohydrate *intolerance*. Nutritionally oriented physicians have long known that some people with food intolerance do better on what is termed a Stone Age diet. The milk products and grains we've so recently introduced into our food chain may be hard for some of us to digest. This theory is propounded in a fascinating book called *Food and the Gut Reaction*, by Elaine Gottschall (Kirkton Press, Ontario). Gottschall proposes that chronic bowel problems, and even such devastating conditions as Crohn's disease and ulcerative colitis, can often be cured by limiting certain carbohydrates.

The simple theory? Sucrose (table sugar), lactose (milk sugar), and the by-products of incomplete starch digestion (from grains, breads, potatoes, and other starches) remain in the gut and act as food for pathogenic bacteria. These bacteria ferment the food, produce toxins, and inflame the intestinal lining. The lining forms a thick layer of mucus in an attempt to protect itself—thus limiting its own ability to absorb nutrients. A diet limited to simple carbohydrates made of single sugars can dramatically cure these long-standing problems.

Gut toxicity takes three basic forms: candida yeasts, bacteria, and parasites. When candida proliferates in the colon, it probably causes an unseen reaction much like that in a woman's vagina: inflammation, redness, swelling, and a mucous discharge. Candida can, in cases of extremely severe immune suppression, invade the surface of almost every organ in the body, leading finally to candida septicemia, a bloodstream infection. Candida septicemia can be fatal. Elizabeth Taylor told *Life* magazine in an interview that she suffered from just such a candida infection after being cured of her last bout of near-fatal pneumonia, because the doses of antibiotics given her were so high and her immune system so devastated by the severity of the pneumonia. By the way, this almost never happens in immune-competent individuals, so don't worry that if you are given antibiotics for a routine infection you'll invariably end up in such a dire situation.

Nevertheless, candida infection can begin in the gut and travel up the GI tract to the stomach, the esophagus, and finally the mouth, where it appears as a white coating called thrush. Candida produces what are known as *endotoxins* (internal toxins). When these toxins are concentrated and rubbed onto the skin of human volunteers, an irritating rash appears. Clearly, these toxins can damage the tissue of the gut. The inflamed wall can become more porous, letting the toxins through into the bloodstream. Even undigested food particles can pass through the gut wall—and if they float into the bloodstream, the body treats them as foreign invaders and manufactures antibodies. This may lead to food allergies, or hypersensitivity reactions to common foods.

The end result? Fatigue, malaise, and a constant feeling of being unwell.

A toxic gut can also be a home to *parasites*. When you think of parasites, your first image may be the dense rain forests of Africa or South America. But recent research has shown parasite infection to be far more widespread in this country than previously thought. Today, in a world made small by air travel, parasites are international. Food carrying parasite cysts is flown to this country from every remote corner of the globe. Immigrants from tropical and subtropical regions may be carrying parasites. And transoceanic travelers who go scuba diving in the West Indies or trekking through the Amazon jungle bring back these microbes as well. No wonder three out of every five Americans will experience a parasitic infection at some point. Over a million Americans are infected with roundworms and another 20 million with pinworms, and 80 percent of army cadets (in one study) from the West Coast were infected with *Toxoplasma gondii,* another parasite.

How does parasite infection manifest? In its chronic form, it can cause mild bowel disturbances, allergies, and persistent fatigue. I see this kind of parasite-linked fatigue often in my patients.

The most common parasitic infections in the United States are giardiasis and amebiasis. Some studies show that about 10 million Americans are infected with *Entamoeba histolytica* (which causes amebiasis) and another 8 million with *Giardia lamblia.* The symptoms of amebiasis include diarrhea, gas, bloating, fatigue, and malaise. Amebas usually reside in the large intestine.

Giardia, in turn, typically infects the duodenum, in the small intestine. Chronic infection can cause malabsorption, resulting in malnutrition and fatigue. This is particularly serious in the case of giardia, because a considerable percentage of nutrient absorption takes place in this section of the small intestine.

Parasites tend to stimulate the immune system to send in defenders called eosinophils. These cells carry proteins that are toxic to pathogens. They also trigger the release of substances such as leukotrienes and prostaglandins, which cause tissue to become inflamed. Inflammation is like an alarm for the body, notifying it that an area is under attack so it can rush new warriors to the site. The problem is that with

The Inner Environment: Toxins Within

chronic parasite infection, this *inflammation* itself becomes chronic. The gut wall can be damaged.

A third, frequent cause of gut toxicity is bacterial imbalance. Fatigued patients *commonly* harbor an overgrowth of common pathogenic bacteria—such as staph, harmful strains of the normally beneficial *E. coli*, or a bacteria called Klebsiella.

The best way to do an all-round check for yeasts, parasites, and bacteria is a test like the Comprehensive Digestive Stool Analysis from Great Smokies Diagnostic Laboratory (Asheville, North Carolina), or any other reputable laboratory. This stool analysis looks for many common pathogens, along with other indications of bowel toxicity (such as the level of degenerated eosinophils or other by-products of allergy or inflammation). Don't be surprised if the results show a mixed infection—yeasts, parasites, and bacteria may be growing as thick as moss under a wet stone. Once the gut has become toxic, it's easy for new invaders to take hold.

Stool samples taken by conventional doctors usually look only for the presence of parasites—ignoring bacteria and fungus. They know there are as many bacteria in the human intestine as there are stars in the nighttime sky. But a new notion is grabbing researchers in gut and autoimmune diseases: that of *dysbiosis*, or an overgrowth of harmful bacteria. Some of these bacteria are the ones commonly implicated in serious respiratory and bladder infections later in life in immune-compromised individuals.

Parasites, in particular, may require additional tests. These little critters can be extremely difficult to diagnose, since they often cling to and burrow into the gut wall. Standard stool tests are only a "spot" check, and the cysts or adult organisms may be missing from that particular sample. Even several samples taken in a row may not reveal the presence of parasites. The best test is a rectal swab, a painless procedure in which a cotton swab–type applicator is swabbed vigorously in the rectum in order to catch parasites that may be clinging to the gut wall. This test is particularly effective when combined with sensitive new techniques that detect not just the presence of the parasite but of its antigen (a chemical "footprint" that lights up with fluorescent stain). There are also stool and blood tests for antibodies to parasites like amebas.

The good news is that the gut can be detoxified effectively through diet, potent herbs (and sometimes prescription medicines) to kill pathogenic microbes, and cleansing techniques such as fasting and diet modification. Here's the program I recommend to patients:

Shift immediately to a diet low in refined foods, alcohol, and saturated fats. I suggest emphasizing low-fat animal protein, vegetables, and natural fibers—since, as I've noted, pathogenic bacteria, yeasts, and parasites thrive on indigestible carbohydrates. If this diet doesn't provide relief, you may need to restrict carbohydrates to simple-sugar sources (fruits, vegetables, some beans, honey, certain cheeses, and yogurt), as outlined in Elaine Gottschall's book.

It's also important to provide beneficial bacteria in the form of acidophilus and bifidus supplements, and in severe cases, to add natural absorptive clay in the form of bentonite. These products can be obtained in most health-food stores. Think of this approach as improving the ecology of your internal garden.

If possible, have your doctor test the levels of hydrochloric acid in your stomach. This can be done with the Heidelberg Gastric Analysis, an ingenious device that monitors stomach-acid levels without any discomfort to the patient. After fasting for twelve hours (you can simply skip breakfast in the morning), you ingest a small capsule that contains a pH sensor with a tiny transmitter. A belt attached to the Heidelberg machine is worn around your stomach. The machine monitors the path of the capsule through your system, reading levels of stomach acid. If your stomach acid is low, supplement it with hydrochloric acid tablets at every meal. Hydrochloric acid in the stomach is the first defense against parasites.

The next step is to kill the pathogens and replace them with beneficial bacteria. Yeasts can be killed with the prescription drug Nystatin, in powdered form. It is regarded as extremely safe by physicians and is tolerated well by individuals of all ages, even babies. Nystatin is not absorbed outside the gut, but it will kill yeasts from your mouth to your rectum. For those with a more serious yeast problem—yeast and fungi may have settled in the sinuses, the vagina, or the skin—a new systemic drug, Diflucan, is quite effective. This drug was initially developed to help combat the severe fungal infections that seem to attack immunocompromised patients such as those suffering from

AIDS. It worked so well that it has come into general use. It is, however, prohibitively expensive for those who don't have medical insurance (about $9 a pill).

Natural yeast fighters include caprylic acid (a fatty acid that inhibits yeast in the intestines), grapefruit-seed extract (a natural antiyeast and antiparasitic substance), and garlic supplements. After an initial "frontal" attack with prescription medications, patients can often switch to these natural substances to keep the upper hand in the battle against yeasts.

For parasites, I favor natural substances. I find antiparasitic drugs have powerful side effects and are hard for patients to tolerate. Though I will sometimes prescribe these drugs (such as Atabrine and Flagyl), I often prefer to start with two natural weapons: artemisia, an herb that has been proven effective against resistant strains of malaria, and grapefruit-seed extract, a substance that strongly inhibits the growth of parasites. These two substances, when combined, are quite effective in inhibiting parasites. They need to be taken over a period of weeks or months, but they are gentle on the system. Two types I use are Paramicrocidin, a citrus-seed extract, and Artemesinin (from Allergy Research Group).

When there is a serious overgrowth of bacteria, or what we call dysbiosis, I usually prescribe cleansing techniques, along with supplements of beneficial flora. I think of this as a process of internal gardening, rather than dosing someone with powerful "pesticides" that kill off all their flora. I tell my patients their GI tracts are like the once-luxuriant forest of Washington State, where Mount Saint Helen exploded and totally devastated the flora. Specialists estimated it would take three hundred years to reforest totally, and what grew back first were weeds. In order to accelerate the process, forestry experts planted and nurtured seedlings. Now they estimate the forest will be luxuriant again in less than a century.

The "seedlings" for our internal forest are beneficial flora, known as acidophilus and bifidus, which are most effective in powdered, refrigerated form. They are stirred into a glass of pure spring water in the morning, an hour before eating, so that they will pass unharmed by digestive enzymes into the small intestine and colon, where they can compete with other bacteria for space and nutrients. Both acidophilus and bifidus are milk-based, but they come in dairy-free powders for those who are allergic to milk. The brands I prefer are Bifido Factor (Allergy Research Group) and DDS Acidophilus (UAS Labs).

Occasionally, a patient just doesn't get better with supplementation, natural herbal antibiotics, and dietary change. One patient of mine suffered from intermittent diarrhea, allergies, and fatigue. Her bowel test showed an overgrowth of Klebsiella, a pathogenic bacteria that I see commonly in my practice. When I gave her Cipro, a potent prescription antibiotic, for five days, she instantly felt better, and she remained well on supplements of beneficial acidophilus.

I recommend many different cleansing techniques to my patients. For those patients who can tolerate it, I first recommend a few days' fast. However, fasting can be very hard on the body, particularly if you have a blood-sugar problem like diabetes or hypoglycemia. It must be done under supervision and is only a good idea for certain patients. I've seen people who, after being ordered to fast by well-meaning naturopaths, come to my office weak and emaciated. The problem: Many patients with gut dysbiosis also suffer from malabsorption. If the gut wall is inflamed, they may require nutritional supplementation, since all inflammatory diseases cause the body to burn calories while it tries to repair itself. Fasting on just water or juice can deprive such patients further of needed nutrition, and sometimes instead of giving the body a rest, it accelerates the inflammatory process. Fasting is equally hard on patients suffering from CFS, who need to nourish their bodies as much as possible to fight chronic activated viruses.

Some physicians also advise enemas and colonics as a method for cleansing the colon. Though I don't commonly recommend them in my practice, I think they can be helpful under strict supervision. Some practitioners specialize in giving colonics, but I strongly advise that you do this only with your doctor's approval, after having ascertained that you have no serious disease of the colon. Colonics usually cost about $60 a visit. Some patients undergoing a long-term detoxification program prefer to buy a home unit, as it is cheaper and more private. Once again: do not undertake home colonics without a knowledgeable doctor's supervision. Some practitioners even recommend coffee enemas. When taken in this form the coffee goes directly to the bile ducts in the liver (via the portal vein), stimulating them and helping the liver to release stored-up toxins. Other practitioners recommend retention enemas with implants of acidophilus or other beneficial bacteria.

An effective way to clean the gut is to brush it from the inside. This can be done by taking the husks of psyllium, which is a seed that in its refined form is the basis of many fiber supplements, like Metamucil. Ground psyllium seed speeds up the transit time of digested foods through the colon to under twenty hours—instead of the three days many individuals require. One popular formulation is known as Perfect 7, manufactured by Agape Health Products (800-767-4776). Perfect 7 is a gentle formula that contains ground psyllium along with herbs that are known to help lubricate and soothe the gut. It also contains bentonite, a natural clay that adsorbs toxins. Formulations like this can help cleanse the GI tract. Sometimes patients are astonished by what this formula pulls out of their gut—it brushes years of impacted fecal matter off the gut wall, much as a Rotor-Rooter cleans out a clogged drainpipe.

Even gut toxicity is unwittingly recognized by the traditional medical establishment. Doctors treat hepatic encephalopathy—severe liver toxicity—by clearing the gut of toxins. This is done by giving neomycin, an antibiotic that is not absorbed outside the gut. Neomycin sterilizes the entire gut. Then lactulose, a powerful laxative, is given until the patient experiences diarrhea. Together, neomycin and lactulose clear the gut of all toxins. The result? The brain is freed of toxic overload and the symptoms of mental confusion, nightmares, and insomnia often suffered by patients with cirrhosis of the liver are relieved.

Your Energy Plan

Stop taking antibiotics and hormones. Switch to a diet low in sugar, chemicals, and refined food. If symptoms persist, adopt a Stone Age diet emphasizing protein, greens, certain beans, and yogurt, as outlined in the book *Food and the Gut Reaction.*

Get tested for low stomach acid, and take hydrochloric-acid supplements and pancreatic enzymes, if necessary, to improve digestion and help combat pathogenic bacteria.

Supplement your diet with beneficial bacteria in natural yogurts that contain acidophilus, along with supplements bought in the health-food store.

Get a Comprehensive Digestive Stool Analysis, along with a rectal swab, to detect the presence of yeasts, parasites, and harmful bacteria.

If you are suffering from an invasion of gut yeast, switch to a diet low in sugars of all kinds to help starve yeast. Ask your doctor if he will prescribe Nystatin or another antifungal drug to kill the yeast. Also take antifungal supplements like garlic, caprylic acid, and grapefruit-seed extract.

If you are suffering from parasites, confer with your doctor, who may recommend antiparasite drugs or herbs. The latter are gentler on the system but take longer to work. They include, as previously mentioned, Paramicrocidin, a grapefruit extract, and *Artemisia annua*, an antimalarial herb.

If you are suffering from an overgrowth of toxic bacteria, adopt a Stone Age diet, which starves such bacteria.

For all three problems, try Sonne 7 or another intestinal cleanser that contains bentonite (available at most health-food stores), a clay that adsorbs toxins, and psyllium seed, which works like an internal scrub brush to clean the gut wall.

Be patient. It can take many months to cleanse the gut and repopulate it with healthful flora.

8

ENVIRONMENTAL POISONS: YOUR WORLD CAN MAKE YOU SICK AND TIRED

▼

You've looked inward. You've cleaned up your diet, cleaned out your gut, and made sure your endocrine system is working as smoothly as possible. And if you were living in a pristine environment—a mountainside filled with fresh-running streams, nutritious fruits and vegetables, wild game, and clean air—you could probably stop reading this book.

Unfortunately, you're living in the twentieth century. In a world that is, in many cases, toxic.

Eighteen thousand seals washed up dead on the shores of the North Sea in 1988. A thousand dolphins near Spain, France, and Italy died in 1990. Several hundred more dead ones subsequently rolled onto the beaches of Turkey and Greece.

Sometimes, in order to illustrate to my patients the deadly power of environmental toxins, I remind them of these epidemics of the sea. Sea sponges are dying on a large scale. Sea urchins have suffered an epidemic that causes them to shed their protective spikes. Monk seals are becoming extinct.

What is making ocean life die? Scientists speculate that water pollution has weakened the sea creatures, allowing viruses to take hold and utterly destroy the immune system of the animals. They then succumb to myriad diseases. Dead dolphins have been found to harbor up to fifty times the danger levels of toxic PCBs.

Over 150 million tons of toxic waste are dumped into our nation's oceans and rivers every year. But dolphins and whales are not the only vulnerable creatures on this planet. Toxins poison us just as they do the creatures of the sea. Every day, an average of four people are killed by exposure to hazardous substances in this country. Birth defects kill over 8,000 infants a year, cancer kills nearly half a million Americans annually, and scientists suspect that an important cause is environmental contamination. They even have virtual proof in some cases: uranium miners in the Southwest have five times the normal rate of lung cancer.

We have added 60,000 man-made chemicals to our world in the past half century. Not all of us are washing up on the shore, but many of us are swimming aberrantly through our sea of toxins. Before toxic poisoning shows up as cancer or birth defects, it can announce its presence through fatigue. We may be dragging through our days, not even aware that this state of fatigue or grayness is not normal. We forget our birthright of vital, exuberant energy.

Many of my patients find it hard to believe that these invisible toxins may be so intimately linked to their fatigue. They may even wonder if I am leading them astray when I talk about cleaning out poisons through some of the methods in this chapter—from chelating toxic metals out of the body to stripping the home of synthetic carpets, from taking large doses of vitamin C to buying organic wild game instead of your corner butcher's cut of antibiotic-laden beef. I will hear things like, "Dr. Hoffman, I don't see how my carpet can be causing my fatigue. That seems a little farfetched." Not when you have your carpet tested by a specialist who can actually give you a formaldehyde reading, proving that this extremely toxic gas is leaking daily into your home.

We can't always see or feel toxins, but many of my patients respond to our polluted world with vague symptoms of fatigue and malaise that doctors cannot fit into a diagnostic box and give a name to. If you wake up exhausted or suffer from headaches, allergies, depression, and chronic respiratory problems, you may have absorbed toxins from the air and water around you. So bear with me while we go on this journey and take a look at the major sources of environmental toxicity that may be robbing you of vitality.

In this chapter, I will explain the signs and symptoms of environmental poisoning from pesticides, chemicals, and heavy metals. I will

Environmental Poisons

tell you about the array of tests available to pinpoint toxins—tests that most doctors don't know about or use. And I will tell you about all the different and effective ways you can detox. I'll also tell you ways to become "eco-smart" and make your home and office clean.

The twentieth-century world is, in one sense, an assault of toxic chemicals on our body. If you are reading this book in your home or office, chemical solvents and gases are escaping at this very moment from the carpets, glues, and insulation around you. Out in the street you are breathing the chemical exhaust of automobiles. Plastics and synthetic fibers release vapors into your lungs. Modern agricultural methods have exposed you to steadily rising levels of pesticides and herbicides in your meats and produce. These chemicals persist in the soil for years. Your drinking water may be a reservoir for the toxic runoff of waste that has been dumped, both legally and illegally. Your fruits and vegetables contain residues of pesticides, and according to a report issued by the National Academy of Sciences in 1987, pesticides in our food will cause a million additional cases of cancer in the course of our lifetime. For an informative guide to pesticide residues in common fruits and vegetables, take a look at *Pesticide Alert,* by Laurie Mott and Karen Snyder (Sierra Club Books). According to the EPA, 60 different chemicals are used on green beans, 70 on cantaloupes and bell peppers, and 110 on apples. These amounts are typical for many fruits and vegetables.

No wonder that courts have actually awarded compensation to employees who have been "poisoned" by toxic chemicals. In 1988, workers at the Washington, D.C., headquarters of the Environmental Protection Agency actually became ill when new carpets were installed! Some employees went on to develop multiple health problems.

Fatigue is usually the first harbinger of toxic overload: toxins damage cell membranes, disrupt enzyme pathways, and put extra stress on the body as it tries to detoxify and get rid of contaminants.

Though toxic chemicals are not healthful for anybody, each person's body tolerates toxins in varying degrees. There are some individuals who can work directly with a chemical and seem to suffer no ill effects (though the effects may occur twenty or thirty years down the line, with a suppressed immune system that leads to diseases like cancer). Others may become so sensitized or overloaded that they will

WHERE YOU LIVE CAN HURT YOU

▼

Dangerous concentrations of harmful chemicals have been found in some of our country's most beautiful rivers: the Shenandoah, the Chattahoochee, the Mississippi. So-called accidental spills have included a 1988 disaster, where a million gallons of diesel fuel exploded out of a fuel tank in a river near Pittsburgh, poisoning drinking water for more than 800,000 citizens. What did nearby industries do? They took advantage of the wave of toxic oil and dumped their own solvents in as well.

Lung cancer clusters have been identified along the Gulf Coast where—scientists speculate—shipbuilding released asbestos into the lungs of workers. The Mississippi and Ohio rivers both turn out to be deadly streams: deaths from all diseases, including cancer, hug the shores of these two rivers, and are particularly concentrated in counties in the Louisiana delta.

For information on how to make your environment safer, you can contact Greenpeace USA at 202-462-1177, Citizens Clearinghouse for Hazardous Waste at 703-237-2249, or Citizen Action at 202-857-5153.

suffer when exposed to levels so tiny that they are barely detectable even by the most modern technology. Sensitive people appear to reach a "total load," or saturation point, earlier than others. The thing to remember is that these chemical contaminants do not occur naturally in your body.

Although your first impulse may be to hide out in your home, the way primitive people hid in caves to protect themselves from the elements, that may not be a wise idea. Your home could actually be making you sick! The latest battle against pollution has moved indoors to homes and offices, where the average American spends twenty-two hours every day. More than 90 percent of American homes use pesticides, and the Environmental Protection Agency's 1990 study of 4,000 homes in Florida and Massachusetts found "common" household pesticides at much higher levels indoors than outdoors—simply because a closed house tends to keep toxins circulating, while they disperse in the open air. As many as 16 million Americans may be sensitive to pesticides. And even when a pesticide is targeted for removal because it is toxic or carcinogenic, it often takes up to eight years to pull it off the market.

Similarly, offices and "tight" buildings (buildings without adequate air circulation) can pose a pollution hazard. For instance, in 1980 a new high school was opened in Oakland, California, and students and teachers reported difficulty breathing. The problem was eventually traced to the library and storage rooms, in which books were shelved on particle board. The particle board was releasing formaldehyde into the school's inadequate ventilation system.

Indoor pollution levels can be up to 100 times higher than outdoors. Researchers at the Environmental Protection Agency have suggested that indoor pollution may be responsible for over 10,000 deaths each year. And the World Health Organization has concluded that up to 30 percent of new or remodeled buildings are plagued by indoor pollution. In the state of California alone, there are 700 "sick" buildings reported each year.

One of the most common indoor pollutants is formaldehyde gas, which is released from countless materials, from imitation woods, particle board, synthetic curtains, and carpeting. Constant exposure to formaldehyde can cause serious and even irreversible health problems—from extreme tiredness to acute rashes to dry, burning throat and nose, sinus infections, cramps, spasms, urethritis and vaginitis, headaches, and memory loss.

Formaldehyde. Radon. Asbestos. Mothballs. Dust. Poor ventilation. How can you determine if your home is "sick"? There are actually "doctors" who "cure" homes—individuals who specialize in ridding homes of their toxins. One firm, Safe Environments, which has branches in California, will test a house for internal pollution. They'll come to your home with air-quality monitors, gas and radon detectors, and analytical tools for testing formaldehyde levels, electromagnetic fields, and more.

In Manhattan, I use a service called Eco-Buster (they can be contacted through my office). The name is no coincidence—they "bust" the ghostly toxins that can cause illness. This home testing service makes use of the resources of a large company called RCI, which is a Dallas-based environmental company. The cost is relatively modest, considering it can help pave a new road to health and well-being: about $400 for a typical apartment or small home. You get the results in a few weeks.

RCI also sells a kit that allows you to test your water, air, and soil for pesticides, at home, at a fraction of laboratory costs. The kit detects a wide variety of common pesticides.

If you believe you may be suffering from exposure, what can you do? Direct testing of blood levels won't help much. I've tested many patients for toxic levels of chemicals and pesticides, but only one—a man who worked with lacquers—recently showed extremely high blood levels of a toxic substance. His levels of the chemical toluene were 60 times the allowable "safe" levels. No wonder he was tired.

Most patients show "normal" blood levels, but I believe that toxicity may occur at levels far below the official detection limit. Another possibilty is that toxins are sequestered in the fat—but to do a biopsy you need a large-bore needle and a significant amount of fat, and I don't perform that test lightly because it is uncomfortable.

However, there are certain chemical markers of overexposure. For instance, if the urine contains hippuric acid, it's likely there is a problem with formaldehyde. That's because hippuric acid is a by-product of formaldehyde breakdown. I sometimes test for that. I also test for mercaptopuric acid, a by-product of detoxification. When the body is detoxing vigorously, mercaptopuric acid will be in the urine. Similarly, levels of another acid, glucaric acid, show whether the liver is working overtime to metabolize toxins.

For patients who are sensitive to sulfites—which are present in wines and are sprayed on some fresh vegetables to preserve them— the urine can be tested for sulfites. Individuals who have a problem with sulfur metabolism are thought to be more susceptible to Parkinson's and allergic diseases. A mineral called molybdenum can strengthen the pathway that eliminates sulfites.

I also test for antibodies to chemicals. Toxins not only poison you, they can engender a genuine allergic response, in which the blood carries antibodies that can be measured.

Specific chemical sensitivities can be measured by skin tests, or by challenges with actual vapors or gases in a sealed booth. The amount of pentane in the breath can be measured as an indication of free-radical activity in the body.

One possible outcome of chemical exposure is a syndrome called multiple chemical sensitivity (MCS). It has also been called twentieth-century illness, universal reactor syndrome, and environmental illness. The syndrome has a wide range of symptoms: fatigue, flulike symptoms, mental confusion, and all kinds of skin, urinary, joint, and muscle problems.

The chemicals that can provoke this disorder are almost limitless, from the formaldehyde in new clothing to pesticide residues, passive cigarette smoke, lacquers, plastics, and more. In many cases people can trace their illness and sensitivity to a single and overwhelming exposure to a chemical.

One fifty-year-old suburban patient of mine joined her husband on a Sunday afternoon for a relaxing game of golf. All the golfers looked up as a small biplane sprayed pesticides over a nearby fruit orchard. The crop duster then flew over the golf course, but the spray stream was not shut off. A mist of pesticide rained down out of the blue summer sky, engulfing the golfers in a glistening drizzle of pungent-smelling chemicals. Afterward, they went on with their game. The next day, my patient woke up feeling tired and achy. She thought it was the flu, but it didn't go away. A few days later, the smell of her familiar laundry detergent made her so dizzy she had to sit down, and the following week, upon leafing through a women's magazine with a scent-strip advertisement, she developed a severe migraine. (Her husband, in contrast, was fine—his system was able to detoxify the chemicals without being overwhelmed.) We tested her for sensitivity to various pesticides and put her on a six-month detoxification program that included internal cleansing, a clean diet, and removing pesticide residue from her home.

Another patient, an elementary school teacher, stopped by his classroom before Labor Day to do some paperwork. Entering the building, he was assaulted by late summer heat and the odor of fresh paint and newly laid floor tile. He tried to open the windows, but the workmen had carelessly painted them shut. So he braved the near-suffocating August heat and humidity and the fumes of paint in order to complete his first lesson plan. Two hours later he left. Over the next few days, he had difficulty focusing. A trip to a furniture store left him weak and nauseated. His weakness and fatigue worsened, to the point where he had difficulty leaving the house. His doctor thought he was suffering from panic attacks and referred him to a psychologist.

Sometimes toxins give rise to such strange symptoms that they sound like a tale from the realms of science fiction. One professor poisoned by formaldehyde described his extraordinary ordeal in a journal called *Perspectives in Biology and Medicine* in 1991. Philip Klubes was a healthy fifty-two-year-old professor of pharmacology at George Washington University Medical Center when he developed itching on his face and neck. His symptoms gradually worsened over the year, until his eyes began to sting whenever he read books, he felt faint while reading Xerox copies of papers, and he experienced burning pain and stinging on his face just by walking past a shelf of books. Carpets, felt-tipped pens, shopping malls, subways, self-service gas pumps, and permanent press pants: all provoked stinging, burning, coughing, pain, and weakness. He began to smell a terrible stench whenever he was near books or papers. He was diagnosed as having developed a sensitivity to formaldehyde, which is used in processing of paper and countless other items. Eventually he learned that a vent in his small, windowless office had been closed at the time he began to develop his symptoms. His system had been poisoned, and could not detoxify the extra formaldehyde, so that even the faintest whiff of the chemical overloaded him. By wearing a mask and gloves and removing all books and papers from his vicinity, he was able to improve slowly over the next few years.

People with chemical sensitivities are believed by many physicians to be suffering from a purely psychosomatic disorder—their fatigue and strange reactions are often thought to be signs of deep depression. It's hard for doctors to believe that such a wide range of extremely low levels of chemicals could cause so many different symptoms. In particular, fatigue is such a vague "symptom" that almost no conventional doctor is going to link it to exposure to minute amounts of environmental toxins. Yet the Department of Housing and Urban Development recognized MCS as a genuine disability in 1990, and there are bills in both the Senate and House to identify MCS as a health consequence of indoor pollution. Because there have been so many complaints about new carpets (including a case where two men died while gluing down carpet in a closed boat), the Carpet & Rug Institute has agreed to conduct a large study on carpets and their harmful chemical emissions.

Unfortunately, this prominent cause of illness and fatigue has gone largely unrecognized by modern medicine. In 1989, the American College of Physicians issued a position statement calling the relationship between MCS symptoms and chemicals or foods "unproven." In a much ballyhooed study Donald W. Black at the University of Iowa College of Medicine found that "many of the patients in whom chemical sensitivity syndrome was diagnosed were likely to be depressed, anxious, obsessive-compulsive, or to display some other mental ailment. It's clear just from talking with some of them that they had ordinary depression." Other doctors who treat environmental illness were outraged: in a *New York Times* article covering the subject, Leo Galland shot back, "Being sick tends to make people depressed." He contended that people with environmental illness should be compared with others who have chronic diseases.

If your house is sick, how can you clean and cure it? It may be that nature has the best filter for indoor pollution: bring the outdoors inside. W. C. Wolverton, a former researcher at NASA, claims that common houseplants are able to absorb harmful gases and chemical compounds. A two-year study found that plants like English ivy and golden pothos removed significant amounts of benzene, formaldehyde, and other toxic gases in enclosed chambers.

Air filters can also help. Fiberglass air filters are the most commonly available. However, according to physician Joseph D. Sacca, the fiberglass particles (which can cause severe irritation) shed easily—invisibly coating surfaces in the home. To clean air, it's safer to buy filters with activated carbon granules to remove chemicals and gases.

If your water has detectable levels of pesticides or lead, you can buy water filters that will remove toxic chemicals. Many are available on the market; some are easily installed on your countertop, while others are installed beneath the sink. Carefully review their claims to be sure that they filter out lead, copper, bacteria, algae, and chlorine.

Shower filters are also available—and the makers contend that shower water may be more harmful to you than tap water. Standing under the pelting force of a hot shower for fifteen minutes opens your pores, allowing your entire body to absorb chemical-laden water, particularly chlorine. In the body, chlorine can be metabolized into even more toxic chemicals. You can buy shower and water filters from a mail-order service and consulting firm called National Ecological and

Tired All the Time

INDOOR POLLUTION: COMMON CAUSES AND SYMPTOMS

▼

There are countless chemical substances in your home that can cause illness and fatigue. Here are some common ones, and the symptoms that overexposure causes:

Acetic acid is present in certain fabrics and plastics, and as a solvent for gums and resins. It causes irritation of the eyes, skin, nose, and throat.

Acetone is a solvent for oils. It is colorless and sweet-smelling and irritates the eyes, nose, and throat.

Ammonia is a colorless gas that has a pungent smell. It causes irritation of eyes, nose, and throat, as well as chest pains.

Arsenic is used to manufacture pesticides, paints, wood preservatives, and bronze alloys. It causes organ damage and death.

Benzene is a colorless liquid that removes grease and is used in the manufacture of varnishes, lacquers, linoleum, dyes, synthetic leather, and rubber. It's a known carcinogen and damages bone marrow.

Carbon dioxide is a colorless, odorless gas used in fire extinguishers and other chemical processes. Overexposure causes headache, dizziness, elevated blood pressure, and increased heart rate.

Carbon monoxide is a colorless, odorless, poisonous gas in the exhaust of engines, furnaces, and fireplaces. It causes headaches, nausea, weakness, confusion, and sometimes coma and death.

Chlorine is a poisonous gas used in bleaching and disinfecting. It irritates the nose, throat, and lungs.

Formaldehyde is a colorless, pungent gas used to manufacture particle board, plywood, foam insulation, paper towels, grocery bags, household cleaners, and the backs of carpets. It can cause allergic reactions and fatigue.

Hydrocyanic acid is a liquid that smells like bitter almonds and is used in plastics and dyes. It can cause weakness, headaches, confusion, and difficulty breathing.

Lead is a metal used to solder pipes and is present in paint, pottery, china, and machinery. It is toxic to many organs in the body and can poison the brain, nervous system, and blood.

Mercury is a metal used in drugs, fungicides, paints, electrical apparatus, and dental amalgam. It damages the brain, kidneys, and central nervous system, causing a wide range of symptoms.

(continued)

Environmental Poisons

Nitrogen dioxide is a poisonous gas released by gas stoves and furnaces and kerosene heaters. It irritates the eyes, nose, and throat and impairs the lungs.

Paradichlorobenzene is the chemical used in mothballs and is a known carcinogen.

Perchloroethylene is used as a dry-cleaning fluid and solvent. It can injure the liver; cause nausea, dizziness, and fatigue; and irritate the eyes, nose, and throat.

Radon is a colorless, odorless gas commonly found in areas where rocks and soil contain granite, shale, or phosphate. It is the second leading cause of lung cancer, and harmful levels have been found in many homes.

Toluene is a liquid obtained from coal tar and is used as a solvent. It causes weakness, confusion, dizziness, headaches, nervousness, and rashes.

Trichloroethylene is a liquid solvent used in dry cleaning, printing inks, paints, lacquers, and other products. It can cause headaches and fatigue.

Environmental Delivery System (N.E.E.D.S.) (800-634-1380). The company will customize filters for your home if necessary. And finally, water-purification units for your pool, or for country wells, that don't use toxic chlorine are now available. Contact the Withers Mill Company, P.O. Box 347, Hannibal, MO 63401 (or call them at 800-223-0858). These Solarcide filters use silver and copper in a technique spawned by NASA space-age technology to clean water without corrosive chemicals.

You can also substitute nontoxic cleaners for those you are presently using. Some tried-and-true methods:

• Freshen air in refrigerator, closet, garage, storeroom and basement with an opened box of baking soda, activated charcoal, and borax solution.

• Use white vinegar or borax in warm water to clean away molds and disinfect household surfaces.

• Use olive oil to buff shoes. Use beeswax or olive oil to polish furniture.

NATURAL PEST CONTROL

▼

What if your home is overrun by ants, cockroaches, fleas, flies, termites, or spiders? You don't want to share your bed with bugs, but killing the little critters with toxic chemicals can burden your system as well. Here are some ways to control pests without poisoning yourself:

Ants: Sprinkle powdered red chili pepper, dried peppermint, or borax where ants enter. Plant mint around the outside of the house to drive them away.

Cockroaches: Mix baking soda, boric acid, and powdered sugar, and spread around the infested areas. You can also mix oatmeal with plaster of paris. Either mixture will kill roaches. Put bay leaves in infested cabinets, as it will repel roaches.

Fleas: Feed your pet brewer's yeast tablets or powder—it contains B vitamins that cause natural odors that fleas abhor.

Flies: Buy or make sticky flypaper made of a mixture of boiled sugar, corn syrup, and water. Hang cloves, or put citrus oil in the room to repel flies.

For all types of pests, you can buy ultrasonic pest repellers. One popular one is called Deci-Mate, and is carried by the Sharper Image stores.

• Use 1 cup baking soda and 1 cup white vinegar to flush and clean drains.

Saunas and steambaths can help you detoxify—something the Finns have known for centuries. L. Ron Hubbard, the controversial founder of Scientology, was one of the first to develop centers that specialize in detoxification. I've read accounts of patients who, when they detoxed, literally exuded dyes and chemicals through their skin. Magnified photos showed the toxic materials swelling out like tooth-paste from their pores.

Saunas must be accompanied by rehydration. In general, hydrating your system by drinking a lot of pure water can help cleanse your system. It also helps to refresh yourself with an "oil change"—switching to olive and flaxseed oils instead of animal fats.

Herbs that are blood cleansers can help the lymph system detoxify: these include chaparral, burdock root, juniper berries (for the urinary tract), and echinacea. Skin brushing—a popular service at many luxury spas—is another therapy that can help stimulate the lymph system to detoxify. Simply buy a natural-bristle bath brush at a health-food store, and dry-brush your skin along the length of your arms, legs, and body to stimulate circulation and the lymphatic system.

The old notion of sunshine, exercise, and fresh air—the nineteenth-century-sanatorium approach to degenerative illness—is also important to keep in mind. Russians still send their sick to large healing resorts on the Black Sea.

Detoxification must be done carefully and under a doctor's supervision. The toxic burden of some patients is enormous. I'm loath to initiate a strict detoxification regimen with an extremely toxic patient: I liken it to a speeding express train hitting a brick wall. Slow detoxification, over a period of many months or a year, may be easier on these patients.

I must admit that I've scared some patients away with detoxification regimens. When you first withdraw from your addictions—such as caffeine, alcohol, and fatty and sugary foods—and begin to cleanse your body, toxins are released into the system at a fast rate. It can be extremely uncomfortable—causing joint and muscle pains, severe headaches, skin rashes, and nausea. Something like this happens with chelation of lead, particularly in children—the lead pours from its storage places in the cells and is incompletely eliminated by the body. It circulates back into the brain and nervous system. Some doctors now avoid this by administering DMSA, an oral chelating agent available by prescription, along with EDTA, to keep the lead from redepositing in the brain.

The methods of detoxification I recommend are simple and effective. They also require dedication and time, and initiate a slow, steady process of self-healing. As a result most medical doctors don't recommend them. Many doctors don't even believe that toxins can build up in the body and cause disease. Yet the medical profession has its own high-tech methods of detoxification. Dialysis, for instance, is a form of detoxification for patients whose kidneys function too poorly to filter blood-borne waste products.

Heavy Metals

The three most common and toxic heavy metals that can poison our systems and lead to fatigue and illness are lead, mercury, and cadmium. A simple and accurate method of determining toxic levels of these metals is hair analysis—a method that has its detractors but that I feel is a good general gauge of metal poisoning. While not 100 percent reliable, it provides a convenient, inexpensive screening test for toxicity. The very people who decry hair analysis will admit that hair is actually a roughly accurate indication of levels of toxic metals. I don't guide my tired patients' lives by hair analysis, but if it turns up positive for toxic heavy metals like lead, mercury, and cadmium, I go on to other screening techniques.

One of the most reliable approaches to determining heavy metal toxicity is to *test* a person with a chelator—a substance that tends to pull metals and minerals out of the body. You simply give the person two urine tests—one before chelation and one after chelation. If there's a dramatic increase in metals in the urine, toxicity is almost certain. (By the way, if certain minerals aren't pulled out as well, it means you have a deficiency in those particular minerals. In either case, mineral supplementation during chelation therapy is a must.) Chelation tests can pick up lead toxicity in people who have stored high levels of lead in their bone, even though blood levels may be "safe."

Lead may be the most notorious metal of the toxic triumvirate. Lead laces our soil, water, and crystal. The good news: blood levels of lead declined by over 30 percent between 1976 and 1980, probably because we phased out leaded gasoline and lead paint. Even so, the National Academy of Sciences contends that 600,000 tons of lead is dumped into the atmosphere each year. But experts contend that the biggest danger of lead poisoning continues to be old lead paint, which is still peeling from the walls of 57 million American homes. Most houses and apartments built before 1950 contain lead paint, and until 1977, many brands of paint were laced with lead.

In children, lead poisoning is documented to cause pallor, retching, and listlessness. Even back in the time of Hippocrates, Greek shipbuilders who poured lead into molds for keels would leave work vomiting and delirious. The Centers for Disease Control keep lowering the safe blood levels of lead for children—from 60 to 40 micrograms per deciliter of blood in 1971 all the way down to 30 in 1978, and then 25 in 1985. Now the EPA has proposed 10 as the threshold for damage to developing brains and nerves. Testing of all children has been recommended to be sure their lead levels are safe. I don't know whether *any* levels of this toxic metal are "safe," at any age. The slowing of red blood cell production that can lead to anemia begins at a lead level of 25 micrograms per deciliter—in an adult.

Lead is ubiquitous in our modern, polluted world. The soil in your yard may contain lead, mostly from paint that has peeled off the outside of your house. Water is an extraordinarily common source of lead— mainly because of the lead soldering that joins pipes together. China, porcelain, and other dishes often contain lead in their glazes—but when correctly fired, the lead should be sealed in. However, glaze can begin to leach lead after being exposed to scouring soaps or the acids in fruit juices, wines, vinegars, and coffee. The FDA estimates that 14 percent of imported dishes exceed safe lead limits—and one study of brandy stored in lead crystal for over five years discovered levels of lead soared to over 20,000 micrograms of lead per liter (the safe level in water is 50). Over 1.02 billion lead-soldered food cans hit the shelves of our grocery stores every year, and over 40 million Americans are exposed to lead in their drinking water.

Here is what you can do to protect yourself from lead poisoning. First, test your home with a do-it-yourself lead-testing kit like the Frandon Lead Alert Kit (available by calling 800-359-9000) or Lead-check Swabs (call 800-262-LEAD). These tests are easy to use and will let you know whether dangerous levels of lead paint are exposed in your home.

For guidelines in safely removing lead paint, write to the Alliance to End Childhood Lead Poisoning, 600 Pennsylvania Avenue, S.E., Suite 100, Washington, D.C. 20003. The key to safe removal is not exposing yourself to the dust—and using a special vacuum after renovation that will actually suck up lead dust (regular vacuums spew it back into the air).

To test your water, call the water safety hotline of the Environmental Protection Agency (800-426-4791). Lead contamination is most serious in areas with soft water, which tends to corrode pipes. Studies have shown that most lead is released the first time you turn on the tap in the early morning (or after it has not been used for six hours). Letting the tap run for three minutes to flush out the residue in the pipes will sharply reduce lead levels. Always use cold wate. for cooking and drinking. Hot tap water leaches more lead out of pipes.

To ensure the safety of dishware, don't store food or drink in ceramic, crystal, or porcelain containers. If you're uncertain about a particularly gorgeous piece, have it tested for lead at a laboratory.

To protect yourself from lead in the environment, you can "buffer" your body with other nutrients. Lead blocks calcium metabolism, and calcium is necessary for everything from strong bones to a healthy heart. More than 90 percent of lead is stored in bone. Calcium prevents its deposit in bones and teeth, but vitamin D appears to enhance lead absorption. Low-protein diets increase lead absorption, as does a high-fat diet. Even mild lead poisoning can interfere with iron metabolism. Other nutrients, such as magnesium, copper, chromium, vitamin C, and B vitamins all help protect against the effects of lead by blocking its effects on enzymes.

Here's what you should do if you are concerned about lead levels. Test your water. WaterTest, at 603-623-7400, is well known for lead testing. Get your hair and blood lead levels tested. If either test is suspicious, find a doctor certified in chelation techniques by contacting ACAM, the American College for Advancement in Medicine at 714-583-7666. They can be contacted by mail at 23121 Verdugo Drive, Suite 204, Laguna Hills, California 92653. Ask a certified doctor for a "provocative" chelation test using a substance called EDTA. EDTA is known for its ability to pull heavy metals out of the body and is given by intravenous injection. If significant amounts of lead are released into the urine, undergo chelation therapy with an established and experienced physician.

How does chelation therapy work? An intravenous solution of vitamins, minerals, and the chelator EDTA is prepared. This is infused into the bloodstream through a vein. EDTA leaves the body in the same form by which it entered, but on its way out it chelates metals and minerals from the body. Patients usually undergo between ten and twenty chelation treatments, over a period of weeks or months. Each treatment lasts several hours, during which patients can read or watch a movie.

I've seen patients with mysterious low-level, chronic fatigue feel absolutely rejuvenated after a series of chelation treatments. The spring is back in their walk, the energy back in their lives. Circulation is improved, and the body no longer has to work overtime to carry its load of toxic metals.

Chelation therapy must be performed by an experienced practitioner. Since EDTA is excreted by the kidneys, the possibility of kidney damage is a concern and must be closely monitored. Minerals and nutrients may also bind with the EDTA, so their levels must be carefully checked and controlled through supplementation. Chelation must be done slowly over a period of three to four hours. Too much fluid at too fast a rate might cause an increase in blood volume and a fluid overload, which could be problematic, particularly in patients with serious heart disease. Oddly enough, the magnesium in the chelation bottle might cause the opposite—a drop in blood pressure. That's why all patients must be closely supervised.

To safeguard against possible problems, blood and urine tests are taken before chelation to check kidney function. Cardiac function is evaluated, through a stress test and a noninvasive heart test called an echocardiogram. After every few chelations, bloodwork is repeated. The patient is advised to eat a good meal before the treatment, and blood pressure is monitored before and after each infusion. At least 16 ounces of water must be drunk during the treatment to flush the kidneys.

Many people have high mercury levels because of years of eating tuna and swordfish, which sequester high amounts of mercury in their fat. Another common source of mercury poisoning is your mouth. Is it possible that routine dentistry can turn a human being into a toxic time bomb? Just how toxic to the body is the mercury leaking out of ordinary silver fillings? Mercury toxicity is a very real problem, and I see it in my practice every week. Though not everyone with mercury in their mouth should have it yanked out, there are many patients who, even after medical and nutritional work, simply don't get well. They continue to suffer a variety of bewildering symptoms that are typically related to mercury poisoning—ranging from depression, tiredness, and irritability to bleeding gums, swollen neck glands, burning sensations, diarrhea, irregular heartbeat, headaches, and muscle tremors. Mercury has been shown to depress the immune system, and even if mercury fillings are not the sole cause of fatigue and illness, they can be a significant contributing factor. A little-known fact: the bacteria that cause plaque are able to convert ordinary mercury into methyl mercury, a highly poisonous substance.

In 1987 Sweden acknowledged that mercury fillings were not safe. Yet the war being waged over mercury fillings in this country is so heated that in 1990 it became a violation of the American Dental Association (ADA) code of ethics for any dentist to recommend removing amalgam because of mercury. The ADA protests that mercury is stable when mixed with other metals such as silver, tin, and zinc in a filling. But mercury fillings have never been tested for safety by the FDA, and dentists themselves keep scrap amalgam in an airtight jar. Last year, the EPA banned mercury from indoor latex paint because of the dangers of mercury poisoning, yet the vapor level in a patient's mouth after chewing during a typical meal is sometimes as much as ninety times higher than the vapor level in a newly painted room.

For those who are concerned about toxic metals in their mouth, the first step is to test for harmful levels. People rarely show high blood levels of mercury unless they have been exposed to massive industrial contamination. Otherwise, blood tests are notoriously unreliable—especially since mercury has a high affinity for the body's cells, and is soon absorbed from the blood into the cells. Hair analysis is a more reliable method.

For those of us who don't exhibit high hair levels yet have many fillings and show typical signs of mercury toxicity, there may be mercury hypersensitivity. We can test for sensitivity with a simple patch test, where a tiny amount of mercury is applied to the skin to see if there is a local or systemic reaction.

If you decide to have your fillings removed, realize that the procedure itself can be toxic. Vapors will be released into the bloodstream, and mercury fragments may even be swallowed. Patient and dentist must take special precautions, using barriers and dams in the mouth, and removing the fillings in a precise order, according to the electrical charge on the fillings (fillings with a high-negative charge should be removed first, followed by high positives, and finally neutrals). This is because the body is trying to maintain an electrical balance in spite of these small, electrically charged fillings. Our nervous systems have tried to adapt to these little batteries in our mouths, and they need to be removed in a way that is as gentle as possible.

Finally, about an hour and a half prior to removal of the filling, the patient should receive an injection of EDTA, which will then be circulating in the bloodstream while mercury is being removed. The EDTA will bind with the mercury that is absorbed during the dental procedure.

If high levels of mercury have already been stored in your body's cells, two other chelating agents called DMSA (also known as succimer) and DMPS can help pull mercury out. DMSA is taken orally for three days, and urine is tested before and after. If mercury levels are high, either DMSA or DMPS can be used as chelators. Another chelator, which sometimes causes allergic side effects, is known as D-penicillamine (or D-Pen). In addition, the following nutrients are known to chelate mercury in the body: the amino acid L-cysteine, the antioxidant glutathione, the mineral selenium, and vitamin C. Garlic is high in the sulfurs that help chelate mercury. Selenium, in particular, competes with mercury for binding sites in the cell. The other nutrients grab on to mercury and help the cells release it.

A third toxic metal is cadmium, which is used in many electrical and mechanical appliances, batteries, rubber and plastic, insecticides, photography materials, and semiconductors. Since the beginning of this century, environmental pollution in Europe alone has caused a fiftyfold rise in the concentrations of cadmium in the human kidney— where it is known to cause permanent, irreversible disease, sometimes leading to high blood pressure. Like lead and mercury, cadmium can be measured by hair analysis. Cadmium, however, is harder to chelate out of the body than lead or mercury. It tends to stay put in the cells.

Cadmium toxicity is, unfortunately, a real danger in the industrialized world. One study of nearly 1,700 individuals aged twenty to eighty years living in Belgium (which is the main producer of cadmium in Europe) found increased risk of kidney problems in people whose urine levels of cadmium were high. That's because cadmium is known as a cumulative poison, a poison that builds up in the body over many years, and it accumulates mainly in the kidneys. Actually, since the turn of the century there has been a fiftyfold increase in levels of cadmium in the human kidney. High levels of cadmium may also increase the excretion of calcium. This might possibly have an effect on calcium-related problems like osteoporosis. In addition, the body tends to absorb more cadmium when there is less iron. About 10 percent of the general population of Belgium—and therefore probably of other industrialized countries—suffers from cadmium levels that are high enough to harm the kidneys.

A final, real, but little-understood cause of chronic fatigue is electromagnetic radiation. Robert Becker, a pioneer in the use of electricity to heal badly broken bones, has written two books about low-level electromagnetic radiation. Studies show cancer clusters in populations living near power plants and high-tension electrical power lines, both of which expose individuals nearby to constant electromagnetic radiation. There is also evidence that working with computers and sleeping on waterbeds and under electric blankets increase the chance of miscarriage, because the low-level electromagnetic fields are harmful to human health. Nobody knows yet what effect microwaves, televisions, X rays, power lines, and waterbeds ultimately have on our immunity, but they are a form of pollution that may indeed suppress the immune system. It's best to try and avoid exposure where you can. Home tests for radiation emissions from computers are available from the Radiation Safety Corporation (800-443-0100).

Perhaps the most important measure of toxicity in any form is the health of the liver. The liver is one of the most complex and remarkable organs in your body—and it's unquestionably the key to all detoxification.

Your remarkable liver weighs about four pounds, and it plays a hugely important role in digestion, metabolism, and detoxification. Toxic chemicals, drugs, alcohol, solvents, pesticides, formaldehyde, and herbicides—all are detoxified by the liver. The liver's load is staggering, and its ability to detoxify varies tremendously from person to person. Some of us are exquisitely sensitive to drugs, caffeine, and alcohol, and others are like Rasputin—the diabolical Russian monk who was stabbed, poisoned and shot, and wouldn't die.

Detoxification, like any activity of the metabolism, requires energy. That's why people who are toxic tend to get tired. A recent Italian study showed that many patients who did not have overt, actual liver

---

A NEW CLEAN AIR ACT?

▼

California has a reputation for being the most liberal state in the union, and it is the site of a new quasipolitical movement: chemically sensitive individuals are lobbying for "fragrance-free" zones. Will hospitals, schools, restaurants, and airplanes that now have no-smoking sections soon have no-perfume areas? The National Foundation of the Chemically Hypersensitive, a group with 6,000 members across the country, hopes so. Think of it: you might encounter a guard in the lobby of a building who doesn't ask for your identification but simply sniffs you to be sure you're chemical-free.

Perhaps fragrance activists would be encouraged by the popularity of a new product called the Molecular Adsorber, available in health-oriented pharmacies and stores. This clear container attaches easily to the wall and contains countless little beige pellets that draw offending fumes, contaminants, and lingering odors out of the air. Some of the common odors that get "adsorbed" include perfumes, mothball scent, vinegar, and sulfur compounds.

---

disease suffered from subclinical forms of liver toxicity. The liver was releasing excess levels of ammonia (a by-product of protein metabolism) into the blood, causing fatigue and illness. The most severe version of this kind of liver toxicity is known as hepatic encephalopathy. Patients can't sleep at night or they suffer from nightmares and hallucinations and feel exhausted all day. The cause seems to be excess ammonia.

The good news: The liver is an astonishing organ with a tremendous capacity to regenerate. Even when a large portion of the liver is removed as the result of injury, it can recover in a matter of months. People can survive on a tenth of their liver, because it will carry on the entire liver's work.

The bad news: I see so many people with abnormal liver function that it is shocking. The liver enzymes that become elevated in abnormal tests indicate significant damage. Those tests often miss sluggish, torpid liver function. Studies have shown that mild liver dysfunction related to the contraceptive pill, as well as many drugs and chemicals, doesn't always show up on tests. I find the most sensitive way to test for liver function is the caffeine-tolerance test. Caffeine is metabolized through a major detoxification pathway in the liver. Caffeine is also a simple, easily obtained substance. After giving a patient a dose of caffeine, you wait to see how quickly it is broken down and eliminated from the body by measuring urine levels. If levels of caffeine don't decline quickly, it means the liver is not functioning as effectively as it should.

Another sign of liver toxicity: light-colored stools. They indicate that the liver isn't producing enough bile, and that's just one sign that it may not be functioning well. In addition, allergies, fatigue, sensitivities, general malaise, and premenstrual syndrome can all be linked to a sluggish liver that isn't detoxifying substances vigorously enough.

To help the liver detoxify, a diet low in animal protein and fat helps rest the liver. That's because the by-product of protein metabolism is ammonia, which must be detoxified by the liver. Protein should be obtained primarily from vegetable sources (like beans and grains). Drugs should be avoided—even over-the-counter remedies like acetaminophen and antihistamines.

Often I tell my patients with sluggish livers that they need an oil change—just like a car. I tell them to emphasize monounsaturated oils like olive oil, as well as Omega-3 oils, like those in fish and flaxseed, and to steer away from animal fat and hydrogenated fat.

You should also supplement your diet with herbs that are known to cleanse and protect the liver. The two most important are:

Dandelion (also known as *Taraxacum officinale*). You may know dandelion as a common weed, but herbalists know it as an important cure-all. Its official name comes from the Greek *taraxos* (disorder) and *akos* (remedy). Dandelion has long been used as a liver remedy, as well as a general blood purifier. It is extremely high in vitamins, minerals, and beta carotene (dandelion has 14,000 i.u. of vitamin A per 100 grams, as compared with 11,000 i.u. for carrots). Studies show that dandelion increases the flow of bile, and relieves liver congestion.

Milk thistle (*Silybum marianum*). This common plant contains powerful liver-protecting substances, and its extract is stocked by the National Poison Control Center as emergency treatment for ingestion of poisonous mushrooms (particularly the death angel mushroom). Studies have shown it can prevent and correct liver damage, and it increases the liver's level of an important antioxidant, glutathione, by up to 35 percent, an important aid in helping it detoxify substances. That may be why some experiments have shown that with the addition of milk thistle to the diet, the liver was protected from damage by toxic chemicals. Milk thistle also has been shown to help liver cells regenerate.

Nutrients and vitamins that help the liver detoxify include N-acetyl-cysteine, an amino-acid precursor to glutathione. It's used in cases of Tylenol toxicity in hospitals—for instance, when children swallow the contents of a bottle. Tylenol poisoning is one of the most severe kinds; it can destroy the liver in a matter of hours.

Another amino acid, taurine, helps the liver detoxify chlorine. Pantothenic acid (vitamin B5) helps detoxify formaldehyde.

Vitamin C is also a wonderful detoxifier. It's known as the supreme antioxidant. When your metabolic machinery works hard to detoxify substances, it generates heat as an engine does, and that heat creates by-products known as free radicals. Imagine those free radicals ricocheting off cells like little bullets, damaging DNA, and making the body more vulnerable to infection and cancer. Vitamin C engulfs free radicals like a molecular Pac-Man, so they don't damage the body.

Diet is also important in protecting and cleansing the liver. Saturated fat tends to build up in the liver, clogging it and decreasing bile secretion. Lecithin, which contains choline and inositol, helps protect against this. One high-potency form of lecithin, from Advanced Nutritional Technology, is called Phoschol. Beans are also important, because they contain sulfur substances that boost liver function, including methionine, and amino acid. Beet leaves and beet juice help liver regeneration because of their high content of betaine.

I also recommend trying to buy organic foods whenever possible. One of the biggest sources of chemicals in your body is the foods you eat. Consider the shelves of your typical supermarket. Peanut butter is laced with excess amounts of hydrogenated fat to give it a smooth, creamy consistency. Margarine is made of hydrogenated fats, and many sauces and frozen dinners contain the same hydrogenated oils. These oils damage cell membranes and disrupt cellular communication. Food adulteration, food coloring, and food preservatives are extremely common. Then there are inadvertent toxins in our food supply, such as pesticides in fish that result from toxic dumping in the oceans, lakes, and rivers.

Though many people in government argue that these chemicals

are acceptable at low levels, toxic buildup over the years can be harmful. Studies have shown that food can be produced economically using an organic model and crop rotation, which preserves the health of the soil. The National Academy of Sciences recently found that farmers who apply little or no chemicals to crops can be as productive as those who use pesticides and synthetic fertilizers, and now recommends changing to a method of farming that uses fewer chemicals. The report recommended that the government change policies that have discouraged farmers from trying natural techniques. More than four decades of agriculture have focused on increasing crop and livestock productivity by using huge amounts of pesticides, drugs, and synthetic fertilizers. Well-managed alternative farms use far fewer chemicals and produce as much or more crops and livestock. One 720-acre dairy, cattle, and grain farm in Knox County, Ohio, produced 32 percent more corn and 40 percent more soybeans than the national average—all without using chemical fertilizers or pesticides for the last fifteen years. Not only does natural farming work as well, the study found, but it will spare the environment. Weeds and insects develop genetic resistance to these chemicals, which forces farmers to use ever greater amounts.

There is now a mass movement back to natural foods. Many supermarkets have an organic-foods section, and organic produce is available in scores of health-food stores around the country. Green markets, where farmers sell their fresh, just-picked produce, have popped up like oases in the concrete heart of many cities. Here in New York City when I wander through the local open market on a Saturday afternoon, I feel as if I'm in a remote village. The sounds of traffic fade, and farmers smile as they weigh their fresh, tasty, often organic produce on old-fashioned scales. The food is superb. Most of the meat is in the form of free-range wild game, from venison and rabbit to wild turkey and pheasant. Wild game is lower in saturated fat, and higher in healthful Omega-3 oils.

Soon there may even be national vending machines for water, from a firm called Ecology Speak, International. Prototypes, called the Watering Whole, are already available in resort areas, and instead of sugary, preservative-laden sodas, they offer pure spring water, carbonated or plain, with or without natural flavoring.

If you are interested in finding out more about environmental toxins, you can contact HEAL (Human Ecology Action League, P.O. Box 49126, Atlanta, Georgia 30359-1126 ; phone 404-248-1898), which provides a national support group for people suffering from chemical sensitivities. For an excellent in-depth look at chemical sensitivity, send a check for $10 to *Chemical and Engineering News*, Distribution, Room 210, American Chemical Society, 1155 16th Street, NW, Washington, D.C. 20036.

Your Energy Plan

Realize that your fatigue may be due in part to unseen toxins.

Look indoors first for possible toxic pollution. Check the ventilation system in your home and office. Contact RCI Environmental, at 2701 West 15th Street, Suite 250, Plano, Texas 75075 (214-250-6706) for kits to test your home for contaminants. Find a doctor through the American Academy of Environmental Medicine, P.O. Box 16106, Denver, Colorado 80216 (303-622-9755). Ask this doctor to test you for chemical markers of overexposure. Test for antibodies to chemicals like formaldehyde. Ask for a hair analysis of toxic metals. If either of these turn up positive, try a provocative chelation test. If it is positive, ask for a chelation treatment plan. If mercury levels are high, have mercury amalgam fillings removed by a knowledgeable dentist.

Buy houseplants, air filters, and water filters made with carbon, and other devices for cleaning up the home. Contact National Ecological and Environmental Delivery System (N.E.E.D.S.) at 527 Charles Avenue, Suite 12A, Syracuse, New York 13209 (800-634-1380). Use nontoxic detergents and pesticides.

Supplement your diet with antioxidants and chelators of toxic metals, including: L-cysteine, glutathione, selenium, vitamin C, garlic, vitamin E, beta-carotene, zinc, and sodium alginate (a chelator made from algae). Give the liver a rest by switching to a diet low in animal protein and saturated fat and high in green leafy vegetables and beans. Add liver-protecting herbs like dandelion and milk thistle. Try to eat organic foods, and if you can't give up meat, buy organic meats and wild game—contact U.S. Bison Company Limited at 800-225-7457.

TOOLS TO HELP YOU CLEAN YOUR HOME

▼

Leadcheck Swab: These swabs are about the size of a small ciga-rette, and provide a rapid, easy-to-use, sensitive test for lead on any surface. Each swab is odorless, disposable, and nonstaining. To use it you simply squeeze firmly until yellow appears on the end of the swab, and then rub it on the surface to be tested. Within a minute the swab will begin to change color, indicating whether levels of lead on the surface are dangerous. These swabs can be used for:

• Homes built before 1978, which are likely to have been painted with lead-contaminated paint.
• Dinnerware and crystal. The Food and Drug Administration estimates that one in seven sets of imported lead dishes exceed safe lead limits. Lead may also leach out of crystals, so that wine and other beverages should not be stored in crystal decanters (they can be poured from such decanters).
• Solder. Solder that contains lead is used in many piping systems, and the lead is often leached into the water that pours out of your tap. Running the water for a few minutes helps reduce levels markedly. Lead is also contained in some tin cans (about 4 percent of domestic cans), and particularly imported canned foods.
• Dust and soil. Lead-contaminated dust can be easily inhaled and is a major health threat. Lead can come from falling paint chips on the outside of homes, especially during renovation.

Frandon Lead Alert Kit: This kit is another simple home test for lead; it contains a "leaching solution" as well as an "indicating so-lution." The kit can be used in all of the above situations, as well as on dust.

RCI Comprehensive Kit: This super package is a deluxe test kit that includes samples for testing radon, lead, and other contaminants. You can test your water, air, and soil for dissolved pesticides and have the result in minutes. The test detects a wide variety of common pesticides.

When testing a sample of water, you add an activator solution, as well as a white "detector" disk. To test air, you expose the white disk to air for several hours, then dip it in distilled water and the activator

(continued)

solution. For testing soil, you add an equal weight of soil and water and follow the same procedure as you do for air and water. In each case, if the disk turns a strong blue, there is little or no pesticide. If it remains white, pesticides are present at high levels. Shades in between indicate varying degrees of pesticide contamination.

Using RCI you can also test for radon gas (both short-term and over a three- to six-month period), as well as air contaminants such as ammonia, formaldehyde, and carbon dioxide. At the Hoffman Center we find that the most common problem is formaldehyde.

Nilfisk vacuum: Regular vacuum cleaners don't do much for the allergic person, and sometimes they even spew allergens back into the air, making the problem worse. The Nilfisk vacuum, used by NASA to eliminate microscopic particles and dust, can remove asbestos and lead dust from your home, as well as common allergens. It can collect particles that are 300 times smaller than the circumference of a single human hair. This vacuum costs about $400.

9

MOLDS, MITES, AND POLLENS: COMMON CAUSES OF ALLERGIC FATIGUE

▼

Environmental toxins aren't the only external cause of fatigue. Even more common are allergies caused by substances such as molds and pollens. Countless Americans suffer from allergies, and along with their sniffly noses and stinging eyes, they experience fogginess, spaciness, and fatigue. From pollen wafting on a summer breeze to molds growing on a shady, damp porch, elements of the natural world can wreak havoc in the lives of allergic individuals. And yet there are effective solutions to this extremely common cause of fatigue.

I recently saw a twenty-two-year-old woman who was suffering from extraordinary fatigue, headaches, jitteriness, and inability to concentrate. Rita's doctor thought she might be hyperthyroid, but her tests were normal. Her doctor finally referred her to a psychologist, who concluded she was having severe emotional problems related to work anxiety. Rita admitted that she usually felt sick at work, but on weekends she felt "great."

The catch was that she had held her job for three years, and only when the company had moved to a new building had she started feeling tired and sick. I instantly suspected she was suffering from "sick building" syndrome. I asked her to take mold plates to her office and expose them. When we had the mold plates analyzed, they came back with a total fungus and mold growth "too numerous to count." The predominant fungus was an unusual one that usually grows in the soil but can thrive in damp paper, fabric, and straw. My patient went to her employer armed with this report, and an inspection of the elaborate ducting and ventilation system was made. Large, stagnant pools of water were found in the drain pans, and they were totally blanketed with a heavy overgrowth of mold. Her company then contacted a firm that came in and cleaned the ducts of the entire building's cooling system—where mites, mold, and mildew can accumulate. Once the building's air system was cleaned, my patient's fatigue cleared up.

Mold can be found almost everywhere, and all molds produce spores, airborne "seeds" that cause allergic reactions in many individuals. In fact, a study reported in the *British Medical Journal* found that damp, moldy housing is significantly linked to health symptoms. Nearly 600 adults and over 1,100 children were surveyed, their homes were inspected for dampness and mold growth, and air samples were taken of mold spore counts. Dampness was found in 23.3 percent of the households and mold growth in nearly 50 percent. Adults living in moldy houses had many different health symptoms, and children had wheezing, cough, runny nose, fever, and headaches, and were likely to have medications prescribed.

Here are just a few common molds:

Hormodendrum: It grows on plants, leather, rubber, cloth, paper, and wood. It is one of the most common causes of health problems.

Aspergillus fumigatus: Found in soil, in damp hay, on grain, on sausage, and on fruit. The number one cause of respiratory disease in humans.

Phoma: Grows on magazines, books, and other paper products.

Penicillium notatum: Grows on fruits, breads, and cheese. Mutant strains are used to produce the lifesaving antibiotic penicillin.

Mold growth is stimulated by warmth and high humidity, so it tends to be most prevalent during the hot, humid summer months. Walk into a lovely, lush forest grove, with a damp carpet of leaves under your feet, and you have just entered a veritable mold emporium. Basements, compost piles, cut grass, barns, and wooded areas all are high in molds. Taking a hot shower in an old bathroom can cause the mold count to soar temporarily. But I increasingly find cases like that of Sholom (see Chapter 1) or my patient Rita—where the home or office environment is growing a coat of mold as fertile as a rain forest.

An important point about mold allergy is that it is often related to an overgrowth of candida (see Chapter 7), a fungus that causes cross-reactivity to many other yeasts, fungi, and molds. Once a candida allergy has been triggered in the body, a patient may begin to experience allergies to other common molds without understanding the cause of his cyclical fatigue.

Mold and mildew can be controlled with many different products. Allergy Control Products (800-422-DUST) offers humidity gauges, room air cleaners, dehumidifiers, and electrostatic air filters. They offer vinyl box-spring protectors and face masks. To avoid mold in your home, follow these general guidelines:

• Keep humidity as low as 35 percent if possible but in no case over 50 percent. Measure humidity with a gauge.

• Use an air conditioner or dehumidifier in the summer, and spray the air filter with a mold-killing spray.

• Ventilate your house. Tightly closed houses encourage mold growth.

• Keep refrigerators clean. Empty water pans below self-defrosting refrigerators, and clean garbage cans frequently.

• Make sure tiles, shower stall, tub, toilet tank, and ceiling are regularly cleaned with mold-killing solutions. Do not carpet your bathroom.

• Use a dehumidifier in the basement, and cover the floor with a plastic barrier (avoid carpeting over concrete, since that encourages mold growth).

• Remove carpeting in bedroom and encase mattress in impermeable zippered covers. Avoid foam rubber, which is likely to become moldy.

• Be aware that books, wood paneling, old magazines, newspapers, and wallpaper paste support mold growth. Mold grows well in damp, dark closets. A low-watt light bulb can help prevent mold growth in closets.

• Test tropical fibers in burlap bags, hula skirts, and grass place mats. Kapok and jute, two common tropical fibers, are common reservoirs for mold. Kapok is an Indonesian fiber that is stuffed into life jackets, sleeping bags, cushions, and pillows. One test, by Richard Harris, a Beverly Hills allergist, found that 10 patients out of 59 were allergic to kapok, and 9 were allergic to jute.

• Use a good-quality air cleaner to remove mold spores from the air. Portable units are usually not effective.

• When outdoors, avoid cutting grass and raking leaves. If you must engage in these activities, use a face mask. Try to avoid woods where mold growth on rotted logs is high.

• Use a solution of equal parts of household bleach and water to kill mold. Or buy commercial products such as X-14 in a spray dispenser.

Mold allergy is only one cause of allergic fatigue. Allergies are actually shockingly widespread in today's society. Over 20 million Americans suffer from hay fever. About 10 million are victims of asthma, and another 11 million suffer from skin disorders like eczema, hives, and rashes. Many allergic individuals don't realize that their unusual fatigue, irritability, and mood swings may be due to allergic reactions.

Could simple dust be making you sick, achy, and tired? Dust allergy is one of the most common unrecognized allergies I see in my practice, and like other allergies, it inevitably causes fatigue.

For centuries doctors have thought that something in household dust could trigger allergies, but it wasn't until 1964 that a Dutch scientist discovered the microscopic cause of the problem: the dust mite, a little bug related to spiders and ticks that dines on flakes of human skin in carpets, drapes, bedding, and upholstery and leaves tiny fecal particles behind. These particles are so fine that the slightest gust makes them airborne. Dust mites came into their heyday when the vacuum cleaner was invented: the machine inspired countless families to install wall-to-wall carpets, and the happy mites flourished, burrowing so deeply into carpet fibers that no vacuum cleaner could eradicate them.

The most common reservoirs for dust mites: the bedroom mattress, which provides warmth, humidity, and food. A new generation of dust mites can be produced every three weeks. Since most people spend eight hours a day in the bedroom, it is important to miteproof your bed. Mattress, box spring, and pillows should be encased in zippered, dustproof covers.

You can test for the presence of dust mites in your carpet with a kit from ALK, which attaches to the end of your vacuum (from ALK

Laboratories, Inc., Indoor Allergen Analysis Laboratory, P.O. Box 200, Spring Mills, Pennsylvania 16875-9988). A dust sample can be collected by vacuuming for a few minutes, emptying the dust into a petri dish, and then sending it out for analysis, which will determine the mite count and the type of mite. If levels are high, a mite-killing formula can be left on the rug overnight and vacuumed up the next day. One available formula, called Allergy Control Solution, contains tannic acid (commonly found in coffee and tea). The tannic acid doesn't kill the bugs, but it chemically alters their fecal droppings, rendering them nonallergenic.

Dust, molds, foods, chemicals, and pets know no calendar. They can cause allergies at any time of the year. However, if you suffer from seasonal hay fever or allergic asthma, you have probably come to dread the seasons that bring new life and hope to the outdoors. You are already well aware of the havoc pollens can wreak on your life. Not only does your nose get stuffy, or your bronchial tubes constrict, you wake up groggy, and you drag through the day. Think of the familiar image of the allergic sufferer: dark circles under red, itchy eyes, a runny nose, and a dragging, slow walk.

For the hay-fever sufferer, spring, summer and early fall are a nightmare. Grasses, weeds, flowers, and trees send forth their messengers. In March, the American elm shakes out its pollen. In April the sycamore, birch, oak, ash, walnut, and hickory trees follow with high pollen counts. Soon after comes grass, the allergy sufferer's bane. Then comes ragweed, a late-summer arrival.

I am not going to go into great detail about pollen allergy here, as it has been written about so much elsewhere. Two of these books are *Alternate Approach to Allergies*, by Theron Randolph, and *Is This Your Child?: Discovering and Treating Unrecognized Allergies*, by Doris Rapp. I will say that even without overt symptoms such as a runny nose or a wheeze, pollen allergies can cause vague distress and constant, low-level fatigue.

There's an effective solution for most mold and pollen allergies. For more than forty years, many allergy specialists and environmental physicians have used a safe and effective technique to stop allergic reactions. I've referred to it in the chapter on food allergy: it's called neutralization therapy. It doesn't rely on drugs such as antihistamines,

Tired All the Time

COULD ALLERGIES BE CAUSING YOUR FATIGUE?

▼

Ask yourself the following questions. If you answer yes to most of them, you may be suffering from dust allergies:

1. Do you feel worse indoors?
2. Do you feel better outside?
3. Do you feel worse when sweeping or cleaning?
4. Do you feel worse each year when the furnace is turned on?
5. Does your fatigue recur each year with the return of cold weather—when windows are closed?
6. Do you feel worse within thirty minutes of going to bed—as dust particles settle or dust mites on the bed begin to bother you? Or do you feel worse on awakening?
7. Are you worse in a closed-up, air-conditioned home?

If you answer yes to most of the following questions, you may be suffering from mold allergies:

1. Are your symptoms worse outdoors between 5 and 9 P.M., in cool evening air?
2. Do you feel worse in damp places—woods, basement, attics, or certain rooms in the house? Do you feel worse on rainy, gray, humid days?
3. Do you feel worse raking leaves or mowing grass?
4. Do you feel distinctly better after the first late-autumn frost?
5. Do you feel better in an air-conditioned room?
6. Do you feel better when you are away from home or traveling (especially at the seashore, the desert, or high mountain elevations)?
7. Do your symptoms continue beyond the ragweed season (late August)?
8. Are you most improved when temperature is below freezing?

If you answer yes to the majority of the following questions, you probably suffer from pollen allergy:

1. Do you suffer from itching eyes and runny nose?
2. Are you worse outside in the mornings?
3. Are you worse on clear and windy days?

(continued)

4. Are you improved on rainy days?

5. Are your symptoms better inside in an air-conditioned office or home?

6. Do you feel much worse when you go from an air-conditioned room to the outdoors during summer months?

7. Are you improved after the first light frost?

which mask allergy reactions and often leave the user even more tired. It doesn't rely on steroids, which have serious side effects. It relies instead on the immune system itself. By using a very small amount of the allergen—whether it is pollen, mold, chemicals, or foods—the reaction can be turned off. This is a refinement of conventional allergy shots.

Provocation/neutralization is truly an amazing tool, and you have to see it in action to believe it. I've seen one drop of a diluted mold extract cause a patient to start wheezing and sneezing moments later. I've seen children with "behavior problems" who have to be held down by four technicians after a skin injection of an allergen that instantly makes them kick, scream, cry, and exhibit the unruly behavior that made their desperate parents bring them to me in the first place. What's even more magical to see, however, is how rapidly the wheezing, the kicking, screaming, crying, the sudden fatigue—any reaction—subsides when the proper neutralizing dose is given. I've seen people who feel so foggy and disoriented after provocation with an allergen that they can barely write their names but can inscribe perfect block letters a few minutes later after proper treatment.

How does this work? Scientists speculate that the tiny amount of allergen present in the neutralizing dose occupies receptor sites on cells that normally trigger the allergic symptoms. The cells begin to secrete chemicals to turn off the allergy reaction. The signal goes out to the whole body that the allergy reaction has come and gone. A similar phenomenon seems to occur in homeopathy, where double-blind studies have shown that incredibly dilute doses of a substance can neutralize a reaction. Thus, the homeopathic version of poison ivy, Rhus tox, is prescribed to treat skin rashes.

Like a key fitting a lock, the neutralizing dose must be just right—

or the lock won't turn and the allergy reaction won't turn off. Instead, the allergenic dose will further stress the body, causing it to plunge into an even weaker, more fatigued state. That's why a good environmental physician calibrates the dosages very carefully and may work with a patient for hours or days until he finds the proper dose.

When I use this approach in my allergy lab, small, very dilute amounts of an allergen are injected just under the skin of the upper arm. (For certain substances, or where there is extreme sensitivity, drops can be taken under the tongue.) The injection will usually cause both a skin reaction and symptoms that can include itching, flushing, chills, mood swings, dry mouth, stuffy nose, irritability, and sudden, overwhelming fatigue. A typical response: "As soon as you gave me the injection, I felt like crying. My face feels flushed. My hands feel cold. I'm tired."

Successive injections, at either higher or lower doses, will determine the shut-off dose. That proper dose is called the patient's neutralizing dose, and it indicates that the immune system has come down from its hyperactive state to a normal, balanced state.

One caveat: This approach is straightforward, but it can be time-consuming. Each dose of an allergen has to be tested separately every ten or fifteen minutes. The first dilution might be 1:100, the second might be 1:500. If the twelfth dilution is the neutralizing dose, a few hours may have already passed. Though some patients improve immediately on their first visit to the office, others may not improve for weeks.

Once a neutralizing dose is found, a patient can learn how to inject himself at home, or in some cases, drops under the tongue can be used. Both are effective, but I find the drops are better accepted by patients. Tough, recalcitrant cases may require injections. A final, important point that some allergists overlook: as a patient's immune system begins to get back in balance, the dose may need to be changed. Usually it gets higher, or more concentrated, as the patient improves. Patients will know this is happening because mild or moderate symptoms will return. I usually find this happens every three to four months. Some individuals adjust so quickly that they need weekly retesting in the beginning.

Often, allergic patients also need neutralizing doses for histamine, a chemical that mediates all allergic responses and triggers inflammatory reactions. Histamine also functions as a brain neurotransmitter and can profoundly affect mood and well-being. I have often wondered if part of the fatigue and irritability caused by allergic reactions may be due to the effect histamine has on the brain. Patients in my allergy lab have undergone instantaneous and severe mood changes when given a dose of histamine under the skin or under the tongue; neutralizing doses bring them back.

After allergy testing and treatment, I offer my patients an "allergy quencher," an intravenous infusion of vitamin C and other vitamins and minerals known to calm and boost the immune system. Though this intravenous treatment may not be available to you, it is a good idea to take extra vitamin C, which is a natural antihistamine, after an allergic reaction. You can also try a solution of Alka-Seltzer Gold, which can neutralize an allergic reaction. (It is not advertised for this purpose, but it does work through its alkalinizing effect.) Take 1 or 2 tablets and dissolve in a glass of water. Drink it, and then follow with another full glass of pure water.

Your Energy Plan

Test your environment for mold counts by obtaining mold plates from an allergy specialist and exposing them in your home or office.

Take the quizzes included in this chapter to determine the likely cause of your allergic fatigue: molds, mites, dust, pollens.

Have your home examined by a house doctor and cleaned of all possible sources of mold and dust contamination. Buy products that kill mites. Get rid of wall-to-wall carpeting and any old, dusty shelves of books, magazines, or old mildewy wallpaper.

Get tested for sensitivity to molds. Using the provocation neutralization technique, help combat your mold allergies with extremely dilute injections or drops of the molds to which you are sensitive.

Take lots of vitamin C, especially after allergy testing, to help neutralize an allergic reaction caused by histamine release in the body.

10

SLEEP AND RELAXATION: RECHARGING YOUR BATTERIES

▼

Nature has many ways of replenishing the body, but perhaps the simplest and most remarkable is what Shakespeare called "the honey-heavy dew of slumber." It is so obvious, in fact, that lack of sufficient sleep is often overlooked as a source of fatigue.

I emphasize the importance of sleep for three reasons. First, you need a lot of it while you are cleaning out your system and detoxifying, for it allows your body to repair itself rapidly. Second, in this stressful, fast-paced world, deep and restful sleep is a necessity. And third, lack of good sleep is sometimes the central cause of my patients' chronic fatigue. What's even more astonishing is that these patients often believe they are sleeping enough and sleeping well.

Take Rosalyn, a thirty-nine-year-old publishing executive who came to me because she was exhausted and suffered from chronic headaches and sore muscles. She dragged through the days at the office, irritable and depressed, and sometimes she literally pinched herself to stay awake. Even so, in board meetings she occasionally dozed off, her head nodding ever lower until she snapped awake—and observed the quietly embarrassed faces of her colleagues.

She tried to keep herself awake with a lunchtime exercise class, and a nutritious, light meal afterward. It didn't work. By the time she came to my office she had diagnosed herself with chronic fatigue syndrome. But sensitive immunological tests (to diagnose true, immune-related chronic fatigue) came back normal, as did allergy tests and all other measures of health.

Rosalyn's problem turned out to be a lack of sleep—which was a surprise to her. She claimed she was getting eight hours of shut-eye every night. But the clue came from her husband. When the cause of a patient's fatigue seems elusive, I sometimes ask them to come in with their spouse, who can often provide a clue. Rosalyn's husband complained that she snored. Many people who snore sleep poorly.

To find out exactly how well Rosalyn was sleeping, I sent her to an all-night session at a sleep-disorder clinic. Dressed in her blue cotton nightgown, and carrying her favorite pillow, she lay down on a bed in a laboratory and went to sleep with wires taped to her body. During the entire night, she was videotaped and her brain was monitored.

The findings? Rosalyn had a severe case of sleep apnea, or interrupted sleep. Her snoring woke her over two hundred times a night, but she fell back "asleep" so quickly she never remembered waking. Most of her sleep was so light that she rarely had time to get into the deep, restful sleep cycles that we all need. Her snoring would wake her before she had a chance.

About 20 percent of adults snore, but not all of them suffer from sleep apnea. About half of people with sleep apnea have nasal problems, such as a deviated septum, that partially blocks the passageways in their nose. Nasal surgery can correct the problem. Many sleep apnea patients are overweight, and because of the extra fatty tissue in their throats, they have problems breathing at night.

The solution, in Rosalyn's case, proved remarkably easy. A New Jersey orthodontist, Donald Rosenbloom, had invented an antisnore device called Snore Guard. It fitted comfortably into Rosalyn's mouth, keeping her passageways open all night. (For more information, contact Dr. Rosenbloom at 201-845-8411.)

As surprising as Rosalyn's case may sound, it may not be as rare as we might think. A recent, rather remarkable study by Wallace Mendelson and Lauren Krupp, of the Department of Neurology at the New York State University at Stony Brook on Long Island (which now has a special fatigue center), found that sleep disorders may be responsible for a significant number of chronic fatigue cases. Dr. Mendelson is Director of the Sleep/Wake Study Programs at Stony Brook. He and his colleagues saw ten patients who had been diagnosed with chronic fatigue syndrome and who had all the typical symptoms of muscle pain, headache, sore throat, and memory problems. The patients all said their fatigue began suddenly and persisted for at least six months. Nine out of the ten patients had a sleep disorder that was a significant factor in their fatigue.

This study is intriguing, but it doesn't tell us whether sleep disturbance is the cause or the result of an illness. For instance, many chronic fatigue patients have the kind of sleeplessness you have when you're suffering from the flu: sleep is shallow and disturbed. They end up exhausted, and their desperation about their inability to sleep can worsen their problem. I remember suffering from insomnia when I was in junior high school, and feeling fidgety and exhausted in my classes, yet awake and alert at night. The most agonizing aspect of my sleeplessness was that I couldn't foresee any relief from my condition. Some people walk into the bedroom and say, "Thank God, I can't wait to lie down." I approached my bed as if it were a cave of hungry lions. (Medical school cured me of insomnia—I was allowed to sleep so little that I turned into a sleeper of opportunity, able to nod off in chairs and doze through the shattering noise of loud alarm clocks. In fact, medical students get so little time to sleep that New York State recently enforced laws restricting residents' hours to 80 a week. When I was a resident, it wasn't uncommon to have 100-hour workweeks.)

I wasn't alone in my problem, and neither are chronic fatigue patients. Thirty-eight million Americans (17 percent of the population) report that they have trouble falling asleep at night, and 7 percent of us actually rely on medication to fall asleep. Lack of sleep may interfere with health in ways we haven't even calculated. One study of train conductors found that some actually fall asleep while operating the train. And how many drivers doze off at the wheel because of a poor night's sleep? Chronic sleep problems can affect memory, problem solving, and concentration. And insomnia is a significant risk factor in psychiatric illness—and may in fact be the first warning signal of serious depression. Above all, lack of sleep at night leads to fatigue during the day.

Sleep is a universal phenomenon. Every living thing must rest, whether it's the bear hibernating all winter, or the deer sleeping only two hours at a time. Even unborn babies sleep—about sixteen hours a day in the womb. Some scientists believe sleep is a time for the body to repair and balance itself—yet the body also does this while awake.

Sleep is in many ways a mystery. It's like a balanced diet: it occurs in different stages and proportions. It is not just simple "rest." During deep sleep, the body releases most of its growth hormone. Studies show that children with sleep apnea not only sleep poorly, they release less growth hormone and are shorter than their peers. And growth hormone doesn't just make you taller, it's a potent stimulator of the immune system.

A dry medical definition of sleep might be as follows: unconsciousness from which a person *can* be aroused, as contrasted to coma, from which a person *cannot* be awakened. But what happens when we lie in bed unconscious? Are we just passive, dead to the world, stretched out flat for eight hours?

Not at all. Sleep is actually a highly active state. Until the 1930s, most scientists believed sleep was passive, and that in sleep people simply shut down and stopped responding to their senses. Now it appears that sleep is a biochemical web of enormous complexity. The brain must send out chemicals to silence parts of itself and the body. It's as if the brain is in a constant tug of war between a chemical web that keeps it awake and one that keeps it asleep. Cutting a specific part of the brain stem, in fact, leads to a brain that never goes to sleep. Centers deep within the brain stem actively inhibit other parts of the brain and allow sleep to occur.

Older people are told that they simply need less sleep. Unfortunately, the truth is that the quality of sleep tends to ebb with age. Sleep changes with age, and the fact that older people have trouble sleeping could actually be part of the degenerative process of aging. The systems that are actively responsible for arousal and inhibition lose a little of their juice. A thirty-year-old gets only about half as much deep sleep as a twenty-year-old. By age eighty-five, the average person spends about 20 percent of the night awake—though a contributing cause may be that the inactive elderly check in for more sleep than they actually need. And sleep may be more elusive for older people because of the "common" aches and pains associated with aging, as well as emphysema and other respiratory difficulties. Men, additionally, cope with benign prostate enlargement, which causes them to wake and urinate during the night. One study found that 50 percent of healthy people over age seventy have sleep irregularities.

We now know there are two types of sleep, and that during the night these two types alternate with each other. The first is called slow-

---

A CURE FOR INSOMNIA?

▼

Our ultimate cure for insomnia may one day be electrical. If we plant transmitters on strategic places on the scalp and send signals to the brain to regulate sleep centers, we may be able to turn sleep on and off at will. That kind of experiment is actually being done using magnetic devices, at the Scripps Clinic and Research Foundation in La Jolla, California.

Sixty insomniacs held a low-energy electromagnetic device in their mouths for twenty minutes three times a week. Half of them were using a device that actually emitted a magnetic field that stimulated sleep areas of the brain, while the other half were using an inactivated device. Neither group knew which device they had or felt any sensation during the sessions. Insomniacs using the live device fell asleep almost an hour earlier than the other group, and stayed asleep 1.5 hours longer.

---

wave sleep—the deep, restful type of sleep that a person experiences during the first hour of sleep. Though we think of this sleep as the "deep, dreamless" kind, dreams and even nightmares can occur during this sleep. A second type of sleep, called REM (named after the rapid eye movements that occur during this process), happens every hour and a half, and lasts for five to thirty minutes. The dreams that we remember usually occur during REM sleep.

EEG studies of the brain during REM sleep are remarkably similar to waking patterns. That is why REM is sometimes called paradoxical sleep. It seems to be a paradox that a person can be asleep while the brain is highly active. Here are the important hallmarks of REM sleep:

1. Active dreaming—which we may remember—usually occurs during REM.

2. During most REM sleep, a person is usually difficult to arouse. And yet in the morning, when a person awakens, it is often from REM sleep.

3. Muscle tone in the body is deeply relaxed, because of strong inhibiting signals from the brain.

BRAIN WAVES

▼

Whether waking or sleeping, we tend to produce four types of brain waves—and at different times, different brain waves are dominant. They are as follows:

Beta waves: Waves of alert attention that occur between 14 and 50 cycles per second. In beta activity, billions of neurons are engaged in frenetic firing of impulses.

Alpha waves: Waves of relaxation, found in normal adults when they are in a quiet, resting state or meditating, that occur between 8 and 13 cycles per second.

Theta waves: Waves of light sleep or drowsiness, which occur between 4 and 7 cycles a second.

Delta waves: Slow, spindly waves of deep sleep, which occur as slowly as 1 cycle every 3 seconds. This is when heart rate and blood pressure fall and brain temperature actually cools down. Only very adept yogis can generate these waves at will.

---

4. Heart rate and breathing become irregular.

5. Eyes move rapidly, and muscles in the middle ear move.

6. The brain is highly active, and the metabolism of the brain may increase by as much as 20 percent over the normal waking state.

Does the brain actually manufacture a "fatigue" chemical? One study of animals kept awake for several days found that their spinal fluid contained high levels of a special peptide protein. When this protein was injected into the brain of other animals, it caused them to fall asleep almost instantly and stay asleep for several hours. Unfortunately, taking it orally proved ineffective.

Even if we are beginning to understand how we fall asleep, nobody yet knows why we sleep—and why we experience REM sleep. We do know that during REM sleep, signals deep in the brain that would normally cause thought, motion, and activity do not occur. The body and brain are inhibited by sleep, and the overall metabolic rate falls by up to 30 percent. It seems that our body is constantly in a cycle between arousal and rest and that this basic rhythm of existence is reflected in our waking and sleeping. If we stay awake too long, the mind and nervous system begin to malfunction. People can become irritable or even psychotic after being awake for too long.

Skilled meditators know how to replicate the rare patterns of brain waves that occur only in deepest sleep. That rich reservoir of brain rest allows them to do with less sleep and yet to stay biologically "young." During sleep the sympathetic nervous system—the fight-or-flight system—relaxes, and blood pressure falls, muscles relax, and skin vessels dilate, warming the body. The parasympathetic nervous system is more active. This may be why many asthma attacks occur during sleep, when the parasympathetic system causes bronchial tubes to constrict. Asthma sprays can then provide a sympathetic "kick."

The big question everybody asks about sleep usually takes the form of a complaint and it goes something like this: "How come some people can get by on five hours of sleep a night and I need eight?" Why did Albert Einstein confess to needing ten, while Edison relied on short catnaps?

Studies of twins indicate an answer most people don't want to hear: it may be your genetic predisposition. Twins seem to need the same amount of sleep. And though you may get more sleep one night and less the next, your average sleeping time usually remains constant throughout life, except, sometimes, when you are older. Sleeping less is not a behavior that you can learn, and those of us who sleep less than we should are probably impaired at certain tasks during the day.

So, you may wonder, how much should you sleep? Only your body knows the answer: sleep until you feel refreshed. There are a few lucky individuals who are born to be short sleepers. On only two or three hours a night they feel refreshed and energetic. When forced to sleep four hours a night, they feel groggy and irritable.

Insomnia, then, can be defined as the individual's perception of insufficient sleep—sleep that does not leave him feeling restored. Sleeping three hours a night does not define insomnia, if the person in question feels alert and refreshed during the day. Insomnia usually takes the form of:

• difficulty falling asleep (or what researchers call sleep onset difficulty)

- difficulty remaining asleep (sleep maintenance difficulty)
- sleep that doesn't restore (for instance, sleep apnea).

Insomnia can be transient (a few days), short-term (a few weeks), or chronic (a few months or longer). It can have many causes, and just as many solutions. To determine the nature of your insomnia, answer the questions in the chart on the opposite page. Then look for the problem and its solution in the next part of this chapter.

Problems and Solutions

SHORT-TERM INSOMNIA

"Every time I fly to Europe . . . every time my annual report is due . . . every time I sleep in a hotel . . ." Short-term insomnia is easily identifiable, has a specific cause, and lasts a few days or at most a few weeks. It doesn't have a major impact on health or work. One common version is known as "Sunday night insomnia." An individual sleeps late on the weekend, and the sleep cycle shifts slightly so that by Sunday night you don't fall asleep as early as you want.

Solution: By waking earlier on Saturday and Sunday morning, you can easily correct the problem.

DRUG OR ALCOHOL-RELATED INSOMNIA

"A couple of drinks put me to sleep, but then hours later I'm awake." This is a common complaint among drinkers. Alcohol temporarily depresses the nervous system, but it is metabolized rapidly and causes a rebound excitation a few hours later. A person may awake with a start. A lot of people don't realize they have this problem and rely on a nightcap for sleep. (It's the flip side of relying on coffee for energy.)

Solution: Cut out the alcohol. Improvement should occur in a few weeks.

Many drugs can have the side effect of causing sleeplessness—for example, steroids, thyroid hormone, decongestants that contain stimulants, and asthma medications. In addition, nutritional deficiencies due to long-term use of medications can cause sleep problems.

Solution: Drug dosage can be adjusted, or the time of day a drug

DO YOU HAVE A SLEEP DISORDER?

▼

Ask yourself the following questions to determine the possible cause of sleep difficulties.

1. How long have you had trouble sleeping? If only a few days, or even a few weeks, you have a short-term problem. If your sleeplessness has lasted months, your problem is chronic. Short-term problems are usually easier to treat.

2. Does it take you a long time to fall asleep at night? If so, you have a sleep-onset problem. This can often be caused by substances like caffeine and nicotine.

3. Once you fall asleep at night, do you sleep well through the night? If not, you have a sleep-maintenance problem. This can be caused by alcohol, depression, hypoglycemia, or disturbances in your environment.

4. Does your sleep problem cause you anxiety? Could part of the cause of your insomnia be your anxiety? This is known as a psychophysiological sleep disorder. It's as real as any insomnia, but it can be treated through behavioral changes and sleep hygiene solutions (explained later in this chapter).

5. Are you anxious about many things in your life? Do you feel edgy and nervous all day? Your insomnia may be one manifestation of major anxiety or depression. If so, you may need to seek therapy, or even short-term antidepressant therapy.

6. What time do you go to bed? You may be going to bed at a time that doesn't suit your body clock. If so, you could be suffering from a sleep-clock problem. This can be adjusted by changing bedtime hours or by using the same type of light therapy used in certain forms of seasonal depression.

7. What time do you wake up? Perhaps your sleep-clock problem causes you to wake early and feel tired before bedtime. This can also be treated by the same methods mentioned above.

8. Do you sleep late on the weekends? You may be throwing off your sleep clock, causing yourself occasional insomnia.

9. Do you have a changing work shift? Do you work at night? Do you travel across time zones frequently? The body has trouble changing its internal rhythms, hormones, and chemicals when you con-

(continued)

stantly change your time clock. As a result, you may suffer from sleeplessness.

10. Do you take many naps? These could be causing you to stay awake at night.

11. Do you feel refreshed during the day, in spite of lack of sleep? If you feel refreshed, you may simply need very little sleep.

12. Are you feeling sad, blue, down in the dumps? Many depressed individuals attribute these feelings to poor sleep when in fact it's depression that disrupts sleep patterns. The underlying depression must be treated.

13. Does your spouse complain about your snoring? You could have sleep apnea, which causes light, disturbed sleeping patterns that result in constant fatigue.

14. Do you have an achy body? Some light sleepers suffer from an achy body syndrome called fibromyalgia (see page 212).

is taken can be changed. Nutritional and vitamin status should be tested and deficiencies corrected. Quality sleep will often return.

INSOMNIA CAUSED BY CAFFEINE AND NICOTINE

The most common "drug-related" causes of insomnia are not prescription drugs. They are nicotine and caffeine. Caffeine can interfere with sleep up to twenty hours after you consume it. About 80 percent of adult Americans are addicted to a cup of "heavenly" coffee or tea. Caffeine is also present in colas, chocolate bars, and cocoa. Even headache remedies and diet pills contain caffeine. And the truly interesting aspect of caffeine is that it can cause both insomnia *and* sleepiness. I've seen countless patients who had trouble getting out of bed in the morning, until they eliminated their caffeine. In response to caffeine, the body's nerve cells fire more rapidly, giving a feeling of alertness and energy. Unfortunately, a crash must follow the high, and caffeine users interpret that crash as a sign that more caffeine is needed. Finally, the store of neurotransmitters may be depleted and exhausted, and a person may feel perpetually tired. The person may become so accustomed to feeling tired that he assumes it's normal.

Similarly, nicotine can alter your energy patterns, locking you into a constant pattern of stimulation from cigarettes. In addition, cigarette smoke contains high amounts of carbon monoxide, which can impair your tissue oxygenation. Cigarettes, like caffeine, can leave you wired but tired.

Solution: Cut out caffeine and/or smoking. I don't even recommend decaffeinated coffee, because it keeps the taste for coffee alive. Switch to herbal teas or to other energy boosters like ginseng, ginger, and licorice. At night, use calming herbs like valerian, hops, and passion-flower.

CIRCADIAN RHYTHM INSOMNIA

We all have certain inborn circadian rhythms. Our body clock, our temperature, and the fluctuation of certain hormones seem to respond to the rhythm of the day, and of light. In fact, we have a gland in our brain, the pineal, which seems to respond specifically to the absence of light by releasing a hormone called melatonin. Sunlight inhibits melatonin. Darkness lets it flow, and so it usually peaks in our bloodstream at about 2 A.M. When circadian rhythms are forcefully shifted, our body tries to adapt, but it is not always successful. Melatonin production may veer out of control, and the body clock may become so disrupted we have trouble sleeping.

A common form of this that most of us have experienced is jet lag. For the first few days after flying to Europe, we may find ourselves sleepy during the day, and wide awake at 3 A.M. We may feel groggy, disoriented, irritable, or depressed.

Another instance of circadian problems: working the night shift. About 25 percent of American workers have work shifts that are not nine-to-five. The most difficult schedule for the body to adapt to is a changing work shift. The more frequently the shift changes, the harder it is on the body. One patient of mine, a twenty-six-year-old film editor, came to me complaining of exhaustion and depression that was disrupting her entire life. She was working a variable night shift—sometimes from 11 P.M. to 7 A.M., and sometimes from 4 P.M. to 11 P.M. I wrote a letter to her manager requesting that she be given regular hours. When he complied, her symptoms vanished. The coda to the story? The company was bought by another firm, and the new management put her on an irregular shift again. She came back to me complaining of the same symptoms.

Tired All the Time

Even if you aren't flying off to Asia or working the night shift, you may have a profound sleep disorder simply because you're an urban or suburban dweller. You may be suffering from the same disrupted rhythms and light deprivation that a night worker suffers from, because you are constantly working and living under artificial light. The natural cycle of the body seems to be about twenty-five hours. (That's why we get a boost in the fall when we set the clocks back one hour.) Body temperature is lowest in the morning and rises in the afternoon.

Solution: Try to work by day under natural light, in an office with windows. At night, if you are an urban dweller, make sure your shades blot out the light of cities. Allow your brain the peace of total darkness. If you are a shift worker, try to change to an earlier shift. If that's not possible, try to work regular hours.

Melatonin extracts, taken at night, may help regulate the body clock. One study of individuals flying to Europe found that taking melatonin for several days before their flight eliminated much of the impact of jet lag.

Another encouraging new treatment may soon be available for circadian shift problems, and it's simple, safe, and effective. The solution? Expose the individual to light that simulates sunlight. This is a treatment commonly used in treating a form of winter blues or depression known as SAD (seasonal affective disorder). The inner body clock can selectively be manipulated by using bright light.

SLEEP CLOCK PROBLEMS

Early to bed and early to rise, the old saying begins. Another circadian rhythm disorder is linked to "sleep phase." Young people tend to suffer from this problem, where they can't fall asleep at night and can't get up in the morning and are tired all the time except at night. Often this is because of hours kept while in college (late nights and late mornings). Though they may complain of sleep problems, if they happen to go to bed late on a weekend night, they have little trouble falling asleep. Sleepiness may strike them about 2 A.M. after years of training themselves to adapt to late-night rhythms. The typical solution may sound paradoxical: go to bed later and later each night. This "moves" the body clock forward. Each night, the individual must go to sleep three hours later than the night before. It is a hard schedule to follow, but within a week the body clock will have moved up to a reasonable bedtime (say, 11 P.M.).

The opposite problem often occurs in older individuals. They wake up in the early-morning hours completely alert, and feel exhausted in the late afternoon and evening. In other words, they tend to get tired long before their usual bedtime.

Solution: Once again, light therapy may be the new, twenty-first-century solution to the above problems. The prescription: bright, full-spectrum light an hour every evening for those who fall asleep before their bedtime, and bright light an hour every morning for those who can't fall asleep until hours after their regular bedtime. The light now available does not contain UV rays. It is worn in a device strapped around the forehead so that it does not shine directly into the eyes, allowing the wearer to go about normal activities. Contact the National Institutes of Health in Bethesda, Maryland; they have conducted research on light therapy and depression.

RESTLESS LEGS

Some people suffer from creeping, crawling, and aching sensations in their legs, or twitching of the legs that wakes them. This condition is also known as nocturnal myoclonus. One patient of mine slept only one hour a night and complained of horrible sensations of bugs crawling on her legs. She had been inaccurately diagnosed as having a psychiatric disorder. Restless-legs syndrome can be associated with pregnancy, anemia, and other problems.

Solution: Nutritional supplements that help treat and often cure this problem include magnesium, potassium, calcium, vitamin E, and folic acid. Sometimes a patient's requirements for these nutrients can be enormous. One well-educated patient came to me and explained that she had been taking folic acid for restless legs but it hadn't helped. We gave her an intravenous drip with a small amount of folic acid, and her symptoms immediately vanished. However, her oral requirement for folic acid turned out to be *sixty* times the amount in the drip. I often find this to be the case: when a vitamin goes directly to the bloodstream, it can rush to where it is needed. When it must be digested and absorbed, much of it may be lost because of low hydrochloric acid or lack of certain enzymes. Oral supplements, therefore, sometimes need to be extremely high.

BREATHING DISORDERS

Sleep apnea, as has been discussed, is a common cause of insomnia. And sometimes it doesn't result from the patient's snoring. I couldn't solve one woman's sleep problems until I brought her husband into the office and he admitted to snoring. His snoring didn't wake him, but it woke his wife countless times a night. Her sleep was light and disrupted, but in the morning all she knew was that she was tired. She had no memory of repeated waking because of her husband's snoring.

Solution: There are many possible solutions to sleep apnea. If the snorer is overweight, losing weight may help eliminate some of the fat in the throat, thus clearing breathing passages. Cutting out nighttime alcohol and taking an antihistamine or decongestant during allergy season can help. In addition, a new device called Snore Guard (mentioned earlier) that keeps breathing regular is worn in the mouth at night.

When Sleep Is All in the Mind: Problems and Solutions

Sometimes insomnia is related to anxiety about insomnia. An initial period of stress may lead to sleeplessness, and then the sufferer begins to worry about lack of sleep, perpetuating the problem. In this case, it helps to restrict bedtime hours. If a person is sleeping only four hours a night, he can set bedtime hours of 3 A.M. to 7 A.M., for instance. Within two to three weeks, he should be falling asleep more easily, because bedtime is no longer associated with tossing and turning. When he is sleeping more efficiently, he can increase the time in bed by fifteen minutes each night.

Hygiene: An Effective Sleep Solution

If the word "hygiene" sounds like clean sleep, it is. And it is a term commonly used among sleep specialists to indicate setting the conditions for undisturbed slumber.

The first injunction: The more you worry about it, the worse it gets. Even thinking about sleep can cause you to become anxious. Picture the exhausted would-be sleeper, lying in bed with a tensed, rigid body, trying to force sweet sleep to overtake him. It's a contra-

Sleep and Relaxation: Recharging Your Batteries

SLEEP FACTS

▼

• Every nuclear accident reported so far anywhere in the world has occurred on the night shift, when people are tired.

• Most highway accidents take place between midnight and 6 A.M. and are fatigue-related. Their rate is nearly triple that of accidents occurring at noon or 6 P.M.

• People who suffer from severe sleep apnea have more than twice as many car accidents as the general population.

• Fifty thousand car accidents a year occur because drivers fall asleep at the wheel.

• We sleep less now than we did a decade ago, according to data from a Japanese study. In 1970 we slept an average of 7.5 to 8 hours a night. In 1990 we slept an average of 7 to 7.5 hours a night. Nobody knows why this is so, but it may be a result of a faster-paced life, in which we juggle many responsibilities.

• Fifty percent of the elderly suffer from insomnia.

• The average person sleeps 220,000 hours in a lifetime.

• The average healthy sleeper moves forty to sixty times each night.

• Nearly 40,000,000 North Americans snore occasionally.

• The life span of a pillow is supposed to be at least two years.

• Fifteen percent of people sleep in the nude.

• The highest sound level of a snoring sleeper ever recorded is 90 decibels.

• Fifteen percent of children under twelve sleepwalk at least once.

• Louis XIV of France had 413 beds.

• Mark Twain's advice for insomnia was: "Try lying on the end of the bed, then you might drop off."

diction in terms. Sleep cannot be willed. Often sleep needs to be set apart from everything else in life.

• Try to keep your sleep schedule consistent. Plan regular hours of sleep time every day.

• Eliminate caffeine and alcohol, particularly at night.

• Don't exercise or start involving yourself in highly engaging mental tasks near bedtime.

• Don't go to bed hungry or after eating a large meal. Eat a light snack before bedtime or drink a glass of warm milk, which contains tryptophan, an amino acid that is a known sleep inducer.

• Tell your spouse, bedmate, or yourself a relaxing bedtime story. My favorite ones are about my turtle. My wife often asks me to tell her a turtle story, which usually puts her to sleep long before I nod off.

• Take a hot bath.

• Make the bedroom a bedroom, a place to sleep. Don't read or watch TV in bed. Remove all other stimulants from the bedroom, including work and bills.

• Don't nap during the day. Confine your sleep to certain nighttime hours.

As you may have noticed, I've hardly talked about the most common solution to sleep problems: sleeping pills and tranquilizers. As a rule, I don't advocate them. And recently, I felt I was proved right, in the case of the enormously popular drug Halcion. This drug was marketed as a panacea for sleep problems, and while it was helpful in a large number of patients, its side effects (including amnesia, rebound agitation, and short-term memory loss) were so dangerous it was actually removed from the market in England. Now the maker of the drug, Upjohn, has issued stringent guidelines and recommends that the drug not be prescribed routinely for periods greater than ten days. An urgent package insert with these new guidelines has been sent to every physician in the country.

Many physicians are not knowledgeable about sleep disorders, and they have very little time to counsel patients about this seemingly elusive and yet agonizing problem. In some cases the availability of powerful drugs can be deadly: a patient with a major depression may be prescribed a sleeping drug that accentuates the depression and triggers a suicide attempt.

Most hypnotics and sedatives change the nature of sleep. They alter REM cycles and shorten the amount of deep sleep. A person may be "sleeping" eight hours a night after taking a sedative without enjoying the refreshment of natural sleep. That may be one reason many sleeping-pill users complain of being hung over and drowsy the next day. After years of relying on these drugs, a person's health can be damaged in many subtle yet powerful ways.

Your Energy Plan

Take the sleep quiz and determine the nature of your insomnia. If it is *short-term*, take a calming bath, or sleep-inducing herbs like valerian, hops, and passionflower. Drink milk just before bedtime. Don't worry about lack of sleep.

If insomnia is *chronic*, determine possible causes. Follow the solutions listed in this chapter.

■■

EXERCISE: JUMP-STARTING YOUR BATTERIES

▼

The delicious feeling of well-being that results from a truly good night's sleep is matched by one thing: the wonderful exhilaration of an energizing workout. Your body needs both. And these are truly exciting times for people who love to exercise, for we seem to be daily expanding our limits and learning just how great our capacities are.

Until recently, for instance, the marathon was an esoteric athletic event. Only a few ultra-elite specialty athletes ran this grueling 26.2-mile race.

Today, the marathon is so popular it almost seems banal, and the thrilling image of vast hordes of humanity—I participated with over 25,000 contestants in 1991—pounding across the Verrazano Narrows Bridge hardly raises an eyebrow. People in their sixties and seventies train. The marathon is now perceived as so easily within our grasp that it has been apotheosized to the ultramarathon (a race as long as 200 miles), the Iron Man, and even the Double Iron Man—an incredible triple mega-endurance event that includes a 5-mile swim, a 230-mile bike ride, and a 52-mile run. And only recently I heard about a triple Iron Man, an event so rigorous that it is medically supervised. Doctors attend the athletes and give them the go-ahead for each leg of the race. It takes about two days, including supervised rest periods; much of it is performed in states of extreme exhaustion and dehydration. It's the racing equivalent of a fighter on the ropes getting cornered with blows to the head. The winners? Anybody who is not disqualified during the race by a physician.

If just reading about these kinds of races makes you tired, bear with me. What is amazing is not the sheer physical triumph involved but the way we are extending our threshold for stress. One dedicated runner, army sergeant Larry Lovell, remembers finishing a 41-mile trek through the Alps: "When it was over, I sat down and said I'd never do it again. Fifteen minutes later, I was thinking about how I could knock some time off next year."

Statistics show that our records of physical endurance and achievement are continually being broken. Astonishingly, the thresholds of human performance appear to extend and extend. A recent mathematical analysis of the times and records of track and field events shows that if women progress at their present rate they may eventually overtake men—especially in the distance events. Women, in spite of their smaller muscle mass, may have an edge over men in endurance and resistance. They seem to be equipped with a better pain-suppression system, which may be nature's way of helping them through childbirth.

This chapter is not about preparing you for a triple marathon or an Iron Man. It *is* about extending your physical limits and discovering that you can banish fatigue by becoming more active. A walking program can actually boost the immune system in sedentary women, according to a recent study of thirty-six mildly obese, premenopausal women, conducted by David C. Neiman. Eighteen of the women took part in a moderate, fifteen-week walking program, which consisted of forty-five minutes of walking, five days a week. The other eighteen women served as controls. The women who exercised had a 20 percent increase in the levels of certain immune factors in their blood. In addition, those who had upper respiratory symptoms got better in about five days, compared with nearly eleven days for the nonexercisers.

I find striking parallels between the overwhelming stress that endurance athletes face and the stress that causes unremitting fatigue. If we can find out how a trained athlete—working at the limit of his capacity—marshals his body's forces and replenishes them daily, we can apply those methods to everyday tiredness.

Your energy reserves are greater than you know. You may feel now that you're so tired you don't even want to think of exercising. That's exactly how I felt about my first triathlon: impossible! I was in Minneapolis promoting my last book when I called home and my wife said, "You won't believe what I did today. I enrolled you in a triathlon in the Hamptons. The race takes place six weeks from now."

Exercise: Jump-Starting Your Batteries

I was extremely upset. It was mid-July and the race was set for the culmination of the summer. It was both a social and an athletic event. My schedule didn't permit the kind of rigorous training necessary even if I had had more advance notice. But my wife likes to prove to me that I can exceed my limits. And so I trained as well as I could. If I didn't have time to go to the pool, I got on a stationary bike or StairMaster at home. I completed the triathlon, and a year later completed it again in better time—well into the middle of the pack of Wall Street executives, housewives, and born-again jocks.

Whatever your energy limit is right now, you can extend it. In order to do so, you need to familiarize yourself with some basic concepts about exercise. I'll tell you about the distinctly different effects of different kinds of exercise. You'll learn how to monitor your pulse rate and aerobic capacity, and how to incorporate the latest technology to improve your efficiency—and have fun doing it.

There are countless ways to exercise, but only a few different categories. Most exercise can be divided into five types: aerobic, anaerobic, interval (or threshold) training, pulsed exercise, and stretching/yoga. Each type has a different impact on your health, looks, and energy.

The first, and most energizing, is *aerobic* exercise. We might nickname it Energy Exercise—because it is the kind of activity that truly banishes fatigue over time. This is the type of exercise I recommend to almost all my patients. A good aerobic workout leaves you feeling exhilarated and refreshed. It conditions your heart and skeletal muscles, increases the number of mitochondria (the body's tiny energy powerhouses) in your cells, and helps regulate your own internal hormones and natural opiates so that you feel calmer and more relaxed throughout the day. It also increases your energy thermostat, so that you burn more calories.

Aerobic exercise is just what it sounds like: exercise that occurs at a level where oxygen repletion can occur during exercise, so that your muscles remain fully oxygenated. (If exercise continues for a long time, or too strenuously, you cross over into the anaerobic zone. You incur what's known as "oxygen debt." The consequence is accumulation of lactic acid, which causes muscle aches, "burning," and tiredness.) Your muscles, including your heart, burn oxygen for fuel. During aerobic exercise, as your heart pumps quickly, you are flooding your body with oxygen.

Aerobic exercise does not have to be strenuous or exhausting. In fact, you can begin with twenty minutes of comfortable, sustained exercise. Twenty minutes of light exercise a day may indeed be optimal for energy and health. For one person, aerobic exercise may consist of twenty minutes of walking in the woods. For another, it may require strenuous mountain running. The key is continuous, regular exercise. Many people are weekend warriors who play hours of tennis or basketball on a Sunday and hardly exercise during the week. They aren't benefiting their bodies as much as they might think, and they are probably setting themselves up for injury.

Here's a surprising fact: you don't actually accrue a lot more benefit, energy, or cardiovascular health by intense, sustained exercise. It's fun to compete and build your performance level, but if your purpose is to stay in relatively good condition, improve your cholesterol count, and boost your energy levels, twenty minutes a day is adequate. One study, cited by Jim Fixx, the man who began the running revolution in this country, found that a 150-pound person running an eight-minute mile uses 102 calories. That same person running a twelve-minute mile uses 98 calories.

The most important rule? Sense the exertion and feel the challenge, but exercise *within your breath*. The moment you feel breathless, you are performing anaerobic exercise, which is another game altogether. When you feel breathless, begin to slow down. There are many ways of doing aerobic exercise:

Swimming
Walking
Jogging
Cycling
Walking a treadmill
Rowing
Cross-country skiing
Dancing
Aerobic classes

Exercise: Jump-Starting Your Batteries

You may be reading this with a sigh—thinking to yourself, "I know exercise is good for me, and I feel good when I exercise, but I'm just too busy and too tired. When will I ever have time? Besides, I've never been able to keep up a sustained exercise program in my life. Something always happens to throw me off schedule."

I sympathize. The most daunting aspect of exercise is moving from desire to execution. I'm extremely busy, and because I live in the city I can't just walk out my door into a pristine suburban landscape where I can jog at will. And though, like many other New Yorkers, I could join a health club, I might find myself among the nine out of every ten people who join a club and soon stop visiting. (Most health clubs sell ten times as many memberships as they can actually accommodate, because they know that most of their members won't come regularly.)

If you have an extremely busy schedule, why not invest your money in a home bicycle, treadmill, or stair machine? They are available at a variety of prices, depending on their sophistication (see box, page 178). I've found the boom in home exercise equipment a fantastic help. Not too long ago I was standing at the top of my fifth-floor walkup in Greenwich Village watching the shocked and pained expressions of the deliverymen on the day they delivered my 150-pound StairMaster. Now, when I get home at night, I change into my shorts and work out for twenty minutes. It's an energizing and effective aerobic work-out—and the shower is right down the hall.

You may complain that exercising at home is boring, but with the latest advances in exercise technology, even the most monotonous, at-home treadmills are interesting. The newest versions are equipped with elaborate computer programs that alter the speed and the incline of the treadmill. As you run you can watch a screen simulation of the topography you are running on. The new bicycles are also equipped with computer simulations, and you can even buy video tapes to sweep you along the Trans-Canadian Highway or through the alpine course of the Tour de France.

Home exercise has another benefit: for people who are achievement-oriented and like to do two things at once, treadmills and stair machines are an ideal way to catch up on the morning news. Some of my best marathon training was done while watching a good movie on the VCR. Training aficionados might criticize this kind of workout as

---

HOME EXERCISE MACHINES

▼

Richard Miller, owner of the single most popular home gym store in the country, Gym Source, in Manhattan (212-688-4222), says that the three most popular items are treadmills, stair machines, and bicycles. The sophistication of these machines is far beyond what it once was: they contain computerized programs that increase and decrease resistance and show you on a screen exactly what's ahead of you. One popular treadmill, called the Trotter, allows you to create your own program by feeling your way through a workout. As you adjust controls to speed up, slow down, and increase and decrease resistance, the changes are programmed into memory. The machine asks you at the end of every workout if you want to save that particular workout in memory. If so, you'll have exactly the same workout next time. This treadmill costs about $4,000, but some retail for as low as $700. Many stair machines cost about $3,000 but can run as low as $650.

As you might guess, home machines are popular with celebrities. George Bush has a gym, complete with treadmill, stair machine, and weights, built in his suite at the Waldorf, where he stays when in New York City. (The cost? "I can't say," explains Richard Miller. "The government pays for it.") Elton John also has a gym built in his hotel whenever he visits New York, at a price of $15,000 a week. Madonna, Dustin Hoffman, Robert De Niro, Woody Allen, Bill Cosby, and many other celebrities have complete home gyms.

---

low-intensity, and it's true that you may not exercise as intensely while watching *Wuthering Heights*, but a good movie may be just the enticement you need to get you off the couch and onto the treadmill.

An alternative to home exercise is working out at work. Many corporations, both large and small, are now investing in employee health by creating an exercise room. Instead of a traditional two-hour, two-cocktail lunch with burger and fries, employees are encouraged to exercise and take a quick shower and a light lunch at their desk. Not only does their health improve (saving the company medical costs), their lunch hours are shorter as well.

Exercise: Jump-Starting Your Batteries

VIRTUAL REALITY—A NEW UNIVERSE IN EXERCISE?

▼

Imagine watching two people in an empty room that contains a single projection screen. They are wearing wired caps, skintight gloves, and stereo glasses, and they are bobbing, weaving, running. Their gloved hands reach for and catch something invisible in the air. What are they doing?

They are participating in an imaginary world at IBM's Thomas J. Watson Research Center in Hawthorne, New York. Their stereo glasses render the images on the projection screen three-dimensional. They see shapes colliding with each other and the walls. They see those shapes shatter. They are moving in a three-dimensional video game.

It's all part of a new science called virtual reality, a promising field that may revolutionize the way we study, work, and exercise. One day, surgeons-in-training may wield their knives and lasers on simulated patients, while armchair tourists may trek through dense jungles without leaving their living rooms. Virtual reality is already playing a key role in training military pilots: they "fly" in advanced, computer-based flight simulators. Military personnel wage war on simulated battlefields, with simulated tanks that are so realistic they cause motion sickness in new drivers who urge their imaginary vehicles into stomach-spinning capers. Architects use virtual reality to walk on a treadmill while strolling through a visualized, life-size model.

As of today, virtual-reality techniques are primitive—and users must wear bulky instruments and tight-fitting gloves threaded with optical fibers that sense hand movements. But the technology is steadily advancing, and someday we may be able to play tennis at Wimbledon in our den, ski down Alpine slopes in our bedroom, and climb Everest in our own back yard. We may enjoy the delights of thrilling, exotic workouts without ever leaving home.

Another option is to take a night course at a university, and gain access to a well-equipped university gym, with a pool, basketball courts, weight room, and more. The cost is low and the facilities are often excellent.

Finally, if you get bitten by the competitive spirit, you can compete in a wide range of races and become a born-again athlete. Don't think you are too "unathletic," "uncoordinated," or "slow" to compete. Races today are designed for practically everyone, and when you finish a marathon or triathlon, you feel like a hero. The crowd lining suburban streets and standing along curbsides and in parks cheers on the egg-heads as well as star athletes. Anybody who finishes will feel exhilarated by his or her athletic prowess. I like to think of my teammate on the Redline Triathlon Team in New York. Ethel Autorino is sixty-one and raised a family before she decided to take up running in her mid-forties. At the age of fifty-eight she competed in an Iron Man competition. Ethel inevitably surpasses my time at triathlon events by at least half an hour, and at pool workouts this sexagenarian leaves me breathless in her wake.

Moreover, she proves one of the most important facts about exercise: sedentary people who take up exercise later in life will exceed their former life expectancy and experience greater freedom from heart disease. That's not all. Women who are in the highest 25 percent of athletic performance have been shown to have sixteen times less cancer than women in the lowest 25 percent. Exercise even relieves the symptoms of mitral-valve prolapse (MVP), a common heart abnormality. (Women suffering from MVP are often fatigued and suffer from palpitations, anxiety, pain, and dizziness.) When they exercised three times a week, women in one study had a significant decrease in all symptoms and a general feeling of well-being, while a control group had no change at all. In other words, exercise begets health. And health begets energy.

On the other hand, young elite athletes who stop competing in their twenties will find their health on a par with the general population a few decades later. A Swiss study of runners and bobsledders from the national team found that fifteen years later, those who had quit their daily workout were no more fit than a group of men who had never exercised at all.

The cardinal rule of exercise seems to be use it or lose it. I myself have tried it both ways—exercising and not exercising—and there's no comparison. I absolutely cannot achieve high levels of energy and vibrancy when I'm sedentary. I find that I begin to lose my energy in the first month. That's the bad news. The good news is that you can recondition yourself fairly quickly. Even the most sedentary individuals

---

ATHLETES AND AGE: CAN THEY STOP THE CLOCK?

▼

The average age of a major-league baseball player is 28.5 years. Short-stops average only 26.5 years. Pitchers, who only have to stand on the mound and wind up their arm, average the ripe old age of 30. Pitcher Nolan Ryan, past forty, is a monument to the older athlete with his record number of strikeouts and fastballs.

But baseball players are old fogies compared with the stars of some other sports. Female gymnasts peak at age 15, and male swimmers at 20. Sprinters, high jumpers, and long jumpers start to fade at 24. When tennis champion Bjorn Borg made a comeback at the age of 34, he was over the hill—and quickly lost to a little-known Spaniard in about an hour. And when hero Jim Palmer tried to return to the pitching mound at 45, his seven years of rest had slowed his fastball to a measly 75 miles an hour. The major-league average is 88 miles an hour. Knuckleball, anyone?

Still, 75 miles an hour is rather incredible. Physiologists claim that neural and physical regeneration is possible, and that comebacks can occur. Besides, athletes involved in aerobic sports often have long lives. Olympic skiers are known to have a ten- to twelve-year peak period that lasts until the mid-thirties. This year, two cross-country Olympic skiers are 35 and 39. Many female athletes have produced outstanding records after childbirth, including marathoner Greta Waitz. And let's not forget Jimmy Connors, who made a successful comeback at age thirty-nine.

---

will find that within a few months of beginning an exercise program, they are losing weight, eating less, feeling better, and going through their days more refreshed.

How do you determine your ideal rate of aerobic exercise? All of us have a typical resting pulse, which may range from 50 beats per minute to 90 beats per minute. The average is usually in the low 70s. Each of us also has a maximum rate—a speed beyond which our hearts cannot physically beat. Most people's maximum heart rate is about 220 beats per minute—minus their age. Therefore, if you're thirty years old, your maximum heart rate is probably about 190.

One way to determine a "maximum" target pulse range for your aerobic exercise is to use the following formula:

Tired All the Time

1.   Determine your maximum heart rate (220 minus your age).
2.   Determine your resting pulse.
3.   Determine the difference between your maximum rate and your resting pulse, and take 75 percent of that number. If you are more than twenty pounds overweight, smoke, or have recently had surgery or an illness, take only 65 percent of that number.

Your aerobic rate: your resting pulse plus the 75 percent figure above.

Example: A thirty-year-old healthy, fit man has a maximum heart rate of 190. His resting pulse is 70. The difference between those two is 120. Seventy-five percent of 120 is 90. Add 90 to 70 and you get 160. His maximum target should be about 160.

One helpful way to determine whether you are exercising at your aerobic capacity is to buy a pulse meter, a gadget that's becoming extremely popular. It can be worn on the wrist and chest, costs $35–$150, and can be bought in many sporting-goods stores. When I was training for the marathon, I'd run for two to three hours at a time,

---

TARGET PULSE RANGE FOR EXERCISE

▼

When your heart rate hits a certain number of beats per minute, you are exercising *aerobically*. Your breathing may increase, and your breaths may come more rapidly, but you will not feel out of breath. Here are some target ranges: the lower number is the minimum required for aerobic activity, and the upper number is the limit imposed for safety. Keep in mind that condition, weight, and heredity affect these rates.

From age 20–30, your target rate is 145–164 beats per minute.
From age 30–40 your rate is 141–158.
From age 40–50 your rate is 137–153.
From age 50–60 your rate is 133–145.
From age 60–70 your rate is 129–141.

and I wasn't sure how fast I should be running by hour two or three. The pulse meter allowed me to monitor my heart rate and keep it in my aerobic range. I found that at the beginning of my training it was as great an exertion in hour three to run *half as fast* as I did in hour one. Using a pulse meter I was able to sustain my training level at a constant, rather than beginning with a jackrabbit burst of enthusiasm and putting myself into an aerobic "debt" by hour three. And I didn't have to berate myself at the end for dragging along like a tortoise, because I was still hitting my aerobic pace. Gradually, I extended my aerobic threshold.

Another type of exercise is anaerobic. Any exercise that forces your muscles to function in the absence of oxygen is considered anaerobic. When you go for the "burn," you are exercising anaerobically, and waste products such as lactic acid are building up in your muscles and causing discomfort. When you find yourself running breathlessly, you are no longer exercising aerobically. You have stepped into the anaerobic zone, where you are pushing yourself beyond a comfortable capacity. Anaerobic exercise is the type most likely to cause injuries, because you are straining muscles. This is particularly true of sporadic athletes, such as executives whose sole upper-body activity during the week may be turning a key in the lock of their Mercedes, and who hit the tennis court on the weekend for three hours, enduring hundreds of successive concussions (amplified through the length of a tennis racket) along their arm to their elbow. No wonder they suffer from the inflammation known as "tennis elbow." Regular exercise that gradually trains a group of muscles is likely to reduce injury.

Activities like weight training, pushups, situps, and isometric exercises are generally anaerobic. So is any exercise where you push yourself to pain and breathlessness.

Anaerobic exercise does not pay off in quick energy dividends. In fact, it may be fatiguing and depleting, because it overloads your metabolic circuitry. It has its benefits, however. Activities like weight lifting and calisthenics can harden and sculpture your body—making you look good and feel good. Most aerobic athletes include anaerobic exercise in their training regimens because it helps build muscle strength. After you have been exercising aerobically for some time, you may want to add anaerobic exercise to a workout.

• • •

A third type of exercise combines both aerobic and anaerobic training and is known as interval training. It combines steady aerobic exercise with short bursts of high-intensity workouts. It's an optimal way to boost your capacity in a short time. Instead of running for five minutes at a nice, comfortable pace, you run two laps slow and one lap fast. The two laps are within your aerobic capacity, but the fast lap forces you suddenly into the anaerobic zone. It's a challenge that your body seems to adapt to rather quickly, allowing you to upgrade your aerobic capacity faster than usual.

Olympic athletes have recently begun using the bridge between anaerobic and aerobic exercise to create a new kind of workout, known as anaerobic threshold training, which requires that you work out at a pace faster than normal but is not so "anaerobic" and intense that you burn out quickly. Most athletes know the threshold as the point where they begin to tire. By training just below the threshold, they give both heart and muscles a super workout.

How can you determine if you're at your threshold? Exercise at a normal pace, and then push yourself to the point where your breathing becomes labored. Now slow down just a bit so your breathing comes easier, and exercise at that pace for a few minutes. Slow down even more to recover, and once you have recovered, speed up again to just below your anaerobic threshold. Use a pulse meter to pinpoint your threshold.

A fourth, fascinating new approach to exercise is known as pulsed exercise. This was first designed for elite athletes who were under the enormous stress of exhausting daily workouts. But it is also really helpful for people who are so stressed that they are tired all the time. This kind of exercise seems to put them back on the energy map by reconditioning their autonomic (involuntary) nervous system. Invented by vascular surgeon Irv Dardik, who served for seven years as a chairman of the U.S. Olympic Committee's Sports Medicine Council, pulsed exercise has had some extraordinary effects on exhausted patients suffering from everything from multiple sclerosis to chronic fatigue syndrome.

Dardik himself is a whirlwind of energy: a reporter for *New York* magazine described how Dardik followed him into his office but never

Exercise: Jump-Starting Your Batteries

sat down. "Barely pausing for a breath during the next two and a half hours, this tall, broad-shouldered man with curly salt-and-pepper hair and penetrating brown eyes paced my small room and delivered a dazzling lecture." Dardik believes his approach to exercise allows the body, which has become sedentary during illness, to recreate healthy waves of energy that break its own internal, "sick and tired" metabolism. He calls his theory the "Superesonant Wavenergy" theory, and he himself may be the best proof of its efficacy: using it, he recovered completely from a degenerative disease of the spine known as ankylosing spondylitis.

Usually, sick and tired patients are encouraged to spend as much time as possible resting—which may not be good for the body. "Health," Dardik explains, "depends on a balanced relationship between stress and recovery." Exercise, and recovery from exercise, helps create a wave of energy in the body.

Dardik tested this theory with both healthy and ill individuals. He found their resting heart rate, then had them exercise until they hit their aerobic target level and then immediately rest. Healthy patients made a quick "recovery," back to a resting heart rate. Their energy waves were large, responsive, and consistent—somewhat like the odometer surges in a fancy sports car hot-rodding it up the highway. Sick patients had trouble returning to a resting state. Patients with autoimmune diseases found their heart rates climbing even after they stopped exercising. Other patients had difficulty pushing their heart rates up, even when they exercised strenuously. It was as if their autonomic nervous systems had a chaotic, paradoxical response to exercise and rest.

Dardik's approach to exercise for the chronically exhausted (and/ or ill) was to retrain their bodies to make waves. One cycle of exercise and recovery usually takes an individual about three or four minutes. Dardik's patients exercised for *three to seven short cycles* of four minutes, reaching their target rate and then resting. They ran, skipped, jumped, bicycled, rowed, and even lifted weights. Many of his patients with chronic, intractable illnesses and exhaustion made remarkable recoveries using this form of exercise. It was as if their body were retrained to understand the word *recovery*—through pulsed exercise. Then they recovered from their illnesses.

I think Dardik's wave approach to exercise may indeed retrain the nervous system, giving it back the suppleness of response that is the true sign of health. Short bursts of exercise, as well as short periods of recovery, restore the nervous system to synchronization. The fight-or-flight system is once again returned to its original flexible capacity, and the autonomic nervous system is in sync with the demands and stresses of the world. As a result, the body isn't sending out its own eternal "exhaustion" messages in response to constant high levels of stress.

A fifth type of exercise is based on stretching and flexibility. Yoga, which incorporates deep, oxygen-rich breathing exercises and relaxation, is an excellent form of stretching. Yoga masters remain incredibly flexible and strong into their sixties and seventies, performing head-stands and amazingly complex, balletlike postures with ease. A flexible body is youthful and energetic, without the creaking aches and pains of sedentary "old" age. For those who don't like pounding the pavement in running shoes, or working up a sweat in an exercise class, simple yoga postures can help restore energy levels in a peaceful, meas-ured exercise routine. An equivalent exercise from another culture is known as t'ai-chi. Both these disciplines help open up the energy flow in the body.

The nature of all exercise, in our goal-oriented society, seems to be competitive. Whether we are competing with others or with our-selves, we are always trying to enhance performance. That may be why virtually all athletes, coaches, and lovers of exercise (myself included) succumb to the latest promise of a magic elixir that will transform a lackluster performance into an award-winning finish.

To date, there is no such elixir. But there are nutrients that can add an edge to your performance. In addition, nutrients can protect against the kind of free-radical damage that occurs with exposure to oxygen. Exercise floods your body with oxygen, and sometimes free oxygen in the body can cause a process analogous to rusting. This type of cellular damage from exercise is probably minimal, and nutritional supplements can counteract it.

Many regular exercisers on healthy diets are actually deficient in important nutrients. A recent study, reported in the *American Journal of Clinical Nutrition*, found that 60 percent of a group of triathletes were low in zinc and copper, and more than 40 percent were low in magnesium. And 43 percent of female triathletes in this study risked

PULSED EXERCISE

▼

Does exercise make you feel sicker? That's one of the most important questions I ask my patients. A hallmark of deep, chronic fatigue is that when sick and tired patients exercise, they feel worse. (I'm not talking about the regular aches and pains that a sedentary person feels when starting an exercise program.) Patients suffering from CFS who are given a written test before and after exercising will perform substantially worse after the workout. They can become exhausted and mentally confused. They may have a flareup of a viral illness. Exercise does not leave them feeling refreshed—it seems to be just one more added stress on their system.

For those patients, pulsed exercise is like a window of opportunity—a way to recover. One cycle of exercise and recovery takes no longer than four minutes. You must attain your aerobic heart rate and then rest. To vary the muscles used, alternate types of exercise (running, jumping on a trampoline, bicycling, rowing, climbing stairs, swimming).

If you work full-time, try to spend a total of thirty minutes a day doing pulsed exercise. If you're so tired that you can't work, you may be able to perform as many as thirty cycles a day. The middle of the day (between eleven and three) is set aside for a long rest or a nap. Try to alternate a few days of workouts with a day or two of rest.

One typical example of how pulsed exercise helped spur a recovery from chronic fatigue syndrome is the case of Rory Malisoff, a fourteen-year-old tournament tennis player who came down with full-blown CFS—sore throat, swollen glands, headaches, sleep problems, and such enervating fatigue he sometimes stayed in bed all day. When he first began his pulsed exercise program he had trouble getting his heart rate over 100 beats a minute and could only walk for a few minutes before needing to rest. Improvement was gradual but steady, and within a few months he was back on the court.

serious anemia by consuming less than the RDA (recommended daily allowance) for iron. Other studies have found that athletes restricted in vitamins B1, B2, and B6, along with vitamin C, had less aerobic power.

Judging by the tremendous sales of "anabolic" protein shakes—whose brightly colored containers line shelf after shelf in health food stores—one would guess that many athletes have been captivated by the idea that high protein will provide the raw material for muscle growth. Little evidence exists for this. The protein requirements of active individuals may be up to 50 percent greater than that of couch potatoes, but excess, concentrated protein intake can place a strain on the kidneys and liver. Besides, many protein foods are high in cholesterol and saturated fat.

The role of carbohydrates in exercise is less controversial. Carbo-loading, as it's called, boosts performance—which was proven by a study of navy "Seal" recruits. These recruits undergo the most rigorous boot-camp experience in the United States military: they are an elite group of superbly conditioned recruits who are trained for secret reconnaissance missions that may involve covering enormous distances by foot or canoe, subsisting on meager food rations and infiltrating enemy lines. Their regimen causes an anticipated high washout rate. The recruits who survive the training ordeal have remarkable psychological and physical stamina. When navy Seals were put on a high-protein, low-carbohydrate diet, they grew exhausted sooner than men in control groups. Their performance was markedly reduced.

Many athletes actually drink a light, protein-free carbohydrate drink while competing. It can be kept in a water bottle carried in a knapsack or mounted on a bicycle, and drunk before and during a race. A company called Metagenics makes this kind of drink. Known as Endura, it is a calorie-rich solution enhanced with minerals and electrolytes, which are depleted by intense sweating.

By the way, one "aid" most moderate exercisers probably don't need is the so-called sports drinks lining supermarket shelves. Often these drinks contain nothing more than sugar and perhaps some potassium and loads of sodium. You might as well drink a sugary soft drink (to which a generous dollop of salt has been added). The labels of some of these drinks are truly misleading—they often depict someone in the simple act of walking the dog or playing golf. Nobody goes into major sugar debt or electrolyte depletion during these kinds of moderate activities. These drinks, however, have so appealed to the popular imagination that at the Super Bowl we now traditionally pour Gatorade over the winning coach.

Metagenics also makes a protein-and-carbohydrate drink called Opti, which is made to meet the protein demands of intense exercise and can give a much-needed lift. I've found it particularly helpful when switching from one event to another in a triathlon. This drink contains carbohydrate and protein in a predigested, instantly assimilated form, along with a cascade of minerals and vitamins.

Nutrients that elite athletes rely on to enhance performance—and which may help the average exerciser—are called ergogenic aids. Ergogenic literally means energy genesis. These nutrients include:

Dimethyl glycine, also known as DMG, or vitamin B15. DMG gained huge popularity on the training circuit in the 1960s, when it was revealed that successful Russian athletes used this version of vitamin B15 in training. DMG is thought to enhance aerobic capacity and give you a competitive edge.

L-carnitine, an amino acid, has been studied by scientists. It helps shuttle fuel into the mitochondria and is especially low in vegetarian diets, since most carnitine is found in animal tissue. (It can be synthesized by the body but requires vitamin C.) Carnitine is thought to increase something called the VO2 Max, which stands for the Velocity of Oxygen Consumption at Maximum Capacity. To test for VO2 Max, athletes are hooked up to a stationary bicycle or treadmill and exercised to their maximum capacity. At the same time, oxygen consumption is measured with sophisticated laboratory equipment. VO2 Max measures the rate at which oxygen is being used up—and thus reflects the rate at which the person is able to utilize energy. Many new ergogenic aids are measured in terms of their VO2 Max, and carnitine has been shown in studies to increase it.

Octacosanol, an extract of wheat germ, is thought to increase energy and oxygen capacity. Over sixty years ago, nutritionists began to investigate wheat-germ oil, which athletes had long used for energy. After isolating its active energy-boosting ingredient, octacosanol, scientists tested it on athletes. It improves stamina, strength, and reflex reaction time, as well as cardiovascular function. Recent research by Thomas Cureton, director of the Physical Fitness Institute at the University of Illinois, confirms this nutrient's energy-enhancing ability.

Ginseng, also known as Eleutherococcus. The energy-boosting properties of this famous herb may be in part due to the fact that it permits the muscles to release more stored sugar (glycogen) during exercise. The body burns energy more efficiently and recovers more easily. At the same time, ginseng seems to increase the body's burning of fat, and work as an antioxidant, neutralizing free radicals that damage healthy cells. There are many brands of ginseng. One I sometimes use is Ginsana, a standardized extract in a soft, palatable gel.

Choline, a component of lecithin, may be a building block for nerve function, because of a neurotransmitter called acetylcholine. This is certainly true in high-performance athletes. Highly concentrated forms of phosphatidylcholine are available, including one called PhosCol, manufactured by Advanced Nutritional Technology.

Phosphates are sometimes depleted in endurance athletes, and since phosphates are the substances that make up ATP, our energy molecule, they are extremely important. However, the standard American diet tends to emphasize phosphates, which are contained in high amounts in meats and soft drinks. Most of us probably get enough phosphorus in our diet—and too much promotes osteoporosis, especially in women athletes who have so little fat on their bodies (and therefore, have less estrogen circulating in their body) that they stop menstruating. Nevertheless, because of this new interest in phosphates, there has been a carbohydrate "backlash." Some athletes who used to emphasize complex carbohydrates are now putting more animal protein back into their diets.

Tyrosine is an amino acid that helps animals swim longer before becoming exhausted. It's a building block for the neurotransmitters, called catecholamines, that help control the body's response to stress. It's also a chemical precursor to thyroid hormone, which regulates energy.

Your Energy Plan

If you feel too fatigued to start a regular exercise program, consider *pulsed* exercise, utilized by exhausted people often suffering from major illnesses. Try to perform at least thirty minutes of pulsed exercise a day, in four-minute cycles. Exercise until you attain your aerobic heart rate, then rest.

This type of exercise will help reset your autonomic nervous system, taking it out of the cycle of exhaustion and tension and returning it to a healthy cycle of energy and rest.

If you are able to start your own exercise program, begin with moderate *aerobic* exercise. Commit to twenty minutes six days a week—whether it's walking to work, taking the stairs instead of the elevator, jogging in the park, taking a jazz dance class. Make sure to vary your routine to keep yourself interested.

If you are under a time crunch, consider buying *home exercise equipment*. Prices range from moderate to exorbitant; if you can afford them, some of the newest high-tech machines are a pleasure to use. You can also exercise at work; if your company doesn't yet have a gym, talk to your boss about the health and cost benefits (lower insurance costs for the company) of employee exercise.

Once your aerobic program is in place, consider *adding anaerobic* exercise, such as calisthenics or weight lifting, to increase endurance and strength.

If you are inspired, try *interval training* or anaerobic *threshold* training. You may be happily surprised by your own soaring capacity for exercise and energy. Don't be afraid to compete in local races—from minimarathons to triathlons. Remember that folks in their seventies and eighties are doing it!

If muscle tension and stiffness is a cause of your fatigue, try *stretching and breathing* exercises such as those popularized by yoga and t'ai chi. Focus especially on the deep-breathing techniques of yoga, which will flood your body with oxygen.

12

THE DEPRESSION CONNECTION: HOW TO FIND OUT IF MASKED DEPRESSION IS MAKING YOU TIRED

▼

"I felt a kind of numbness, an enervation, but more particularly an odd fragility—as if my body had actually become frail, hypersensitive and somehow disjointed and clumsy . . . There were twitches and pains, sometimes intermittent, often seemingly constant," writes William Styron of his battle with serious, nearly fatal depression, in his memoir, *Darkness Visible*. He could not sleep: "Exhaustion combined with sleeplessness is a rare torture." Finally, Styron admitted himself to a hospital and began to get better. As he concludes, "By far the great majority of the people who go through even the severest depression survive it."

Sometimes the cause of fatigue is not strictly in the body. Even though symptoms may be physical, the source may be hidden depression. Mental attitude is an important slice of everybody's fatigue wheel. An optimistic outlook can help inspire a patient to make lifestyle changes that lead to vitality. That's why I address the possibility of depression with almost every one of my patients.

Depression is not only survivable, it is common. It has sometimes been nicknamed the common cold of mental health—one out of five people will experience serious depression at some time in their lives. In fact, doctors fail to detect signs of depression in about 50 percent of cases, according to the National Institute of Mental Health.

It's very important for physicians to unmask depression. There is increasing evidence that psychological states influence the immune system. Widowers, for instance, have lower numbers of the immune system's infection-fighting cells than do men who haven't lost their wives. And as Norman Cousins noted in *The Healing Heart,* just by thinking of world peace he was able to boost his immune system significantly in twenty minutes—measured by before-and-after laboratory tests!

Perhaps the hardest question I face is the one I ask myself when I am with a chronic fatigue patient, who is sitting there, glum, frightened, world-weary. Which came first, the depression or the fatigue? The answer makes all the difference in my treatment approach. If the primary, underlying cause of their fatigue is depression, why order countless laboratory tests and procedures?

I recently saw a patient who complained of feeling tired, especially in the morning. She complained of achiness and problems in concentrating. After I questioned her, it was clear to me that a large part of her problem was depression. I referred her to a psychiatrist (one sympathetic with nutritional work). Before he could send me an evaluation, the patient returned saying, "I feel so much better. He determined that I was suffering from depression, put me on a medication, and I'm feeling 75 percent improved. I'd still like to know about diet and vitamins, though." On the other hand, doctors often use the psychiatrist as a "turfing" strategy. *Turfing* is a term popular in the lexicon of physicians in hospitals. It's almost a form of gamesmanship in which harried young doctors eliminate patients from their overburdened services by "turfing" them, or passing them to other departments like a football lateral pass. A doctor may seem to be sympathetically listening to your story while his brain is thundering the phrase, "Turf to psychiatry!"

The problem is, the answer is rarely clear-cut. Any chronic illness takes a toll on a person's mood. Moreover, there are certain immune- and nervous-system abnormalities seen in sufferers of chronic fatigue that may actually affect brain chemistry and alter mood. Most of the cases of chronic fatigue that I see and treat have primary physical causes—a hormonal imbalance, a chronic viral infection, allergies. Depression is a side effect of their physical malaise—and in the case of chronic fatigue patients, giving them an antidepressant is akin to spraying perfume on a dung heap. You are simply masking fatigue with a chemical. It doesn't work. Even some psychiatrists who have tried every possible antidepressant on their patients to no avail often are forced to conclude that something physical may indeed be causing their mental state.

But some of my patients are physically sick *because* they are depressed. And it is well known that depressed people are far more vulnerable to physical illnesses. As you will see from the questionnaire below, fatigue and physical ailments are two common signs of depression.

I try to distinguish between fatigue and depression by testing for immune abnormalities, looking for a specific time of onset (a bout with the flu, pregnancy, lifestyle changes), and asking questions about mood. Nonetheless, depression itself can cause immune abnormalities. Studies show medical students, just before exams, have changed ratios of immune cells that are similar to the changed ratios in people suffering from chronic fatigue.

So, even if I conclude that the cause of fatigue is primarily physical, I try to address a patient's mental state. There's no doubt that attitude is an important tool for regaining energy and health.

When a patient's depression is the primary cause of his fatigue and vague symptoms of malaise, I will refer him to a psychiatrist. Often an antidepressant can seem to work miracles, helping a patient quickly regain energy and a new, vibrant perspective on life. But even such cases remain a little mysterious, since certain antidepressants, such as Elavil, also help reduce pain. Elavil, for instance, has been proved effective in some cases of chronic muscle pain (fibromyalgia) and interstitial cystitis (bladder irritation without obvious infection). In the final analysis, we just don't know where to bifurcate physical and mental illness. Besides, depression is as old as time. For tribal peoples, the rite of healing called for a shaman, who danced and sang and sent smoke (the demonic spirit) into the air; for Christians, the ritual of absolution dispelled guilt and sadness, and for many of my patients, the healing ritual that helps boost their mood is the adoption of a healthy lifestyle, a good diet, and exercise.

We all know what depression feels like. Almost no one has escaped the sadness of a friend or relative's death, a divorce or romantic failure, an illness, or a major disappointment. When these things happen we feel empty, tired, and melancholy. But sometimes these feelings of melancholy persist—or seem to plague us for no discernible reason.

COULD YOU BE SUFFERING FROM DEPRESSION?

▼

The following questions are loosely adapted from the Beck Depression Inventory, a classic tool used by psychologists to determine whether a person is clinically depressed. The Beck Depression Inventory is far more detailed and is scored. But these yes-or-no questions will give you a sense of whether masked depression might be a cause of your fatigue:

1. Do you feel blue or sad most of the time?

2. Is your sadness so acute that it feels painful?

3. Do you feel that you have accomplished little that is worthwhile in life?

4. Do you feel you are a failure as a spouse? As a parent? As a friend?

5. Do you feel guilty about mistakes you've made?

6. Are you discouraged about the future?

7. Do you feel bored with life?

8. Do you feel you are being punished, or will be punished?

9. Do you sometimes feel you would be better off dead?

10. Are you irritable much of the time?

11. Do you put off making decisions?

12. Do you cry more than you used to?

13. Have you lost interest in other people?

14. Are you worried that you look old or unattractive?

15. Does it take extra effort to get started at work?

16. Have you lost interest in sex?

17. Do you have little or no appetite?

18. Do you have trouble sleeping?

19. Do you wake up two to three hours earlier than usual and find it hard to get back to sleep?

20. Are you more concerned than usual about your health?

21. Are you constantly aware of aches and pains in your body? And finally:

22. ARE YOU TIRED ALL THE TIME?

The sadness and gloom can deepen until life doesn't seem worth living anymore.

A first bout of major depression most commonly occurs between the ages of twenty-five and thirty, although childhood and adolescent depression are more recognized today as genuine phenomena. Women are three times as likely to become seriously depressed as men, and if you have a relative who has experienced major depression, you are at higher risk. Alcoholics are also at risk for depression.

When people are depressed, they often adopt the behavior of a hibernating bear: they feel tired, they sleep, and they want to be alone. Mild depression can last days or weeks. Major depression drags on for many weeks and months, even years. There are several different kinds of depression:

• **Atypical depression,** which does not always show up as the typical blues. It can also manifest as insomnia, reduced appetite, weight loss, poor concentration, and feelings of guilt. But it can sometimes appear as irritability and anxiety. It may even include voracious hunger and weight gain. Some people with atypical depression feel blue for a few days, then normal for a few days.

• **Bipolar depression,** or manic-depressive illness, includes mood swings from manic excitement and enthusiasm to severe depression.

• **Unipolar depression** exhibits no manic high. A person simply swings from normal behavior to deep depression.

• **Psychotic depression** can mean that the person is not only deeply depressed, but may have hallucinations and hear voices uttering criticism.

No one knows quite what triggers depression, but it is clearly linked to the imbalance of certain brain chemicals, including norepinephrine, epinephrine, dopamine, and serotonin. Antidepressant medications work by regulating levels of these brain chemicals.

There is no doubt that in some cases, antidepressant drugs can be lifesavers—for serious depression is a medical emergency, and appropriate medication can save a life, a family, a career, a marriage.

Antidepressants, unlike alcohol, do not produce immediate results. They usually take several weeks to kick in, and they may initially cause side effects (such as dry mouth, constipation, light-headedness when you stand up). These side effects usually disappear as your body adjusts to the drug.

I personally feel we are relying too heavily on antidepressants, moving toward the brave new world envisioned by Aldous Huxley, where patients buried their negative emotions with Soma, the ideal drug. Take Prozac, apotheosized in a major news magazine that touted this new "miracle" drug for eight pages, and then in the final paragraph raised a serious question: If this drug is so good, is there anyone who isn't a candidate for it? When we get into that kind of thinking we're in danger.

Some researchers are experimenting with the use of bright artificial light to combat depression. Exposure to full-spectrum light—the bulb is worn in a simple headgear device that allows the wearer to go about his or her normal activities—is an effective treatment for depression that is seasonal. This form of depression, known as SAD (seasonal affective disorder), seems linked to levels of melatonin in the brain. Melatonin is a chemical that is suppressed when a person is exposed to bright light. For this reason, some nutritionally oriented physicians are experimenting with the use of pineal gland extract at night to help balance melatonin production and combat fatigue and depression.

Nutrition is an important tool in combating depression. Studies have shown that depression can be linked to frequent consumption of caffeine or sucrose. Research indicates that many people seem to self-medicate their depression with sweets, stimulants, and chocolate. An analysis of the dietary habits of European countries found that the higher the per-capita chocolate intake, the greater the percentage of suicides. Which came first, the depression or the chocolate use? Does chocolate intensify highs and lows of mood? We just don't know.

Deficiencies of various nutrients, particularly the B vitamins and magnesium, are often present in cases of serious depression. Depression is a common symptom when there is a deficiency of folic acid, perhaps because it lowers brain serotonin. Serotonin is enhanced by refined carbohydrates (thus the sugar-addiction connection), as well as by certain antidepressant drugs, including Prozac. B12 deficiency, especially in the elderly, can mimic depression or even Alzheimer's disease. It can be ameliorated with B12 shots.

Vitamin B6 deficiency can be linked to depression, particularly in women. Estrogen blocks vitamin B6, which is required for serotonin production. Therefore, it may be helpful to women who are suffering from PMS, taking birth-control pills, or in estrogen-replacement therapy.

Magnesium is very helpful for atypical, or agitated, depression—where a person is anxious, exhausted, irritable and, deep down, depressed.

Chronic depression, tiredness, and irritability can be part of a subclinical state of scurvy, or vitamin C deficiency. A thousand milligrams of vitamin C daily is recommended. In one study of 885 psychiatric patients, the blood levels of vitamin C were significantly lower than those of healthy individuals.

Other nutrients that can help combat depression include the amino acid L-phenylalanine, or its related form, D,L-phenylalanine. When sixty patients with major depression were given an antidepressant or L-phenylalanine, 30 percent taking the antidepressant recovered, while 60 percent taking the amino acid recovered. When the two groups were placed on a placebo, both experienced a serious relapse.

A related amino acid, L-tyrosine, is also effective. Both these amino acids are building blocks for the biogenic amines—brain chemicals associated with well-being. The discovery of these amines spawned the development of the tricyclic family of antidepressants.

Sometimes a nutritional boost can do wonders for a patient's mental state. My favorite case was a woman whose boyfriend brought her in. Her diagnosis was psychotic depression, and she was living in a halfway house under medication. Her voice was flat, her gaze distant, and her movements mechanical. She seemed to be chemically straitjacketed, and yet her boyfriend insisted that at her core was a creative, loving individual. I took a dietary history and discovered that her meals consisted mostly of creamed corn, chocolate, potato chips, and hamburgers. Her nutritional profile revealed profound deficiencies in beta-carotene, vitamins B6, B1, and C. After supplementing her diet with vitamins and minerals, and modifying it to emphasize greens, fruits, and other more healthful foods, she returned several months later. The dull, lifeless shell of a person had been transformed—I saw an animated young woman, giggling, joking, and bragging about her recent attempts at cooking. Her psychiatrist, recognizing the improvement, tapered her from the most debilitating of her drugs. She was scheduled to leave her halfway house and marry her boyfriend.

Another remarkable case involved identical twin sisters in their sixties. One was robust and rosy-cheeked, the other seemed a shrunken and timid doppelgänger. The healthy sister did most of the talking, while her twin sat in the chair with her mouth twitching in a way reminiscent of a rodent. The story was that she had grown more and more fatigued, had trouble walking, had lost her love of life, and now seemed seriously ill. Her sister felt this was tragic, for they'd always been extraordinarily close, and now she felt a part of herself was dying. A workup by a general practitioner had revealed nothing. My nutritional workup revealed that she was suffering from a severe B12 deficiency, which can derail the nervous system. With her first B12 shot her mouth twitching began to subside, and by her third follow-up visit she was talking and laughing. It took a long series of injections before her walking problems were alleviated.

Depression is common in the elderly, and may often be linked to nutritional deficiencies. Yet an important question this case raised was the role of genetics. Why did one sister suffer from a serious B12 deficiency while the other was healthy? Clearly environment plays an important role, but I recommended to the healthy sister that she have periodic checkups, since she too might ultimately suffer from a B12 deficiency.

You don't have to believe in psychic forces to be fascinated by the mind's power to heal. The new science of *psychoneuroimmunology* (PNI) is focused, as the name implies, on the links between mind, nervous system, and immune system. So far, researchers have found that behavior conditioning can affect the body's ability to fight foreign substances; that nerves from the brain can carry signals to boost immunity; and that brain chemicals also affect the immune system, and vice versa. The new science may explain how someone's belief in a psychic healer—or any other treatment—can speed healing.

The field really began with a groundbreaking experiment by psychologist Robert Ader and immunologist Nicholas Cohen at the University of Rochester. In 1975 they discovered that the immune system could be conditioned, in exactly the same way Ivan Pavlov had conditioned dogs to salivate at the ringing of a bell. Ader and Cohen gave rats a taste of saccharin water and followed it with an injection of cyclophosphamide, a chemotherapy drug that causes temporary illness and also suppresses the immune system. The rats learned to associate saccharin with the drug. And later, when they were given saccharin followed by a harmless injection of salt water, they reacted just as if they had been given the drug again: they got sick and their immune systems were suppressed.

It didn't take long for another research team to show that the mind could also boost immune response. At the National Institutes of Health, scientist Novera Herbert Spector exposed mice to the harmless odor of camphor at the same time that he injected them with an immune-boosting drug. After nine rounds of this treatment, just a sniff of camphor alone increased the potency of the rodents' natural killer cells.

Mind and immunity are clearly linked. The $64,000 question is: How? One exciting and likely answer is that the brain and the immune system speak the same chemical language. One major way nerve cells in the brain send signals to one another is with proteins called polypeptides. The white blood cells, cornerstone of the immune system, also produce polypeptides. These chemicals signal other immune-system cells to produce substances to fight infection. Now it turns out that the white blood cells actually respond to peptides from the brain. And even more exciting, cells deep in the brain respond to the peptides the immune system produces, according to research by J. Edwin Blalock and Eric Smith of the University of Texas at Galveston.

Together, the brain and immune system form a continuous feedback loop, influencing and being influenced by each other. "The immune system is really our sixth sense," Dr. Blalock believes. "It senses those things like viruses and bacteria that aren't recognized by the brain—things you can't see, smell, touch, hear, or taste. The immune system has the ability to convert that information into certain hormones that go to the brain."

The immune system and the nervous system are really much more similar than we have previously realized. Some researchers even believe parts of the two systems may have evolved from the same ancestral cells. As Lewis Thomas has written, the two master systems come together to form "a kind of superintelligence that exists in each of us."

You've probably had the mysterious experience of feeling exhausted and then suddenly getting a "second wind" if something exciting happens. Mood is a subjective aspect of fatigue, and it's a powerful one. Sophisticated scans of the brain called PET (positive emission tomography) show that certain areas of the brain light up when sugar is being used for fuel. The same thing happens when someone is engaged in a mathematical task: dark areas of the brain will suddenly start metabolizing sugar, and they will light up during a PET scan. That means a change in mood or task can instantly "light" up the brain, causing release of energizing neurotransmitters.

Can something as ephemeral as happiness give you energy? Much of the drug industry is based on the premise that we can simply manipulate the chemicals in the brain and thus create a mood of happiness or calm. But can we actually willfully change the way we think and feel—and in that way improve our health?

The answer is a resounding "yes," according to clinical and research psychologist Martin Seligman, Director of Clinical Training in Psychology at the University of Pennsylvania in Philadelphia and best-selling author of *Learned Optimism* (Knopf).

Seligman first became prominent back in 1966, when he developed a novel theory of depression. He claimed that people thought themselves into depression. (And if people can think themselves into depression, they can think themselves into its cardinal symptom, fatigue.) Seligman believed certain people had long ago "learned" to be helpless—just like rats who are repeatedly exposed to painful and inescapable electric shocks and finally stop struggling to get away. Other people were unshakable optimists, comparable to rats who were trained to learn "hopefulness"—these rats were painfully shocked, but they learned that if they pressed a lever, they could stop the shock.

Seligman believed that life experiences could "train" a person, just as electric shock trained rats. He studied what he termed "learned helplessness" for ten years, and his and other studies confirmed a stunning fact: learned helplessness doesn't just affect behavior; it also, in Seligman's words, "reaches down to the cellular level and makes the immune system more passive." Only 30 percent of rats who learned helplessness were able to reject implants of a fatal cancer, while 70 percent of rats who had been taught to master painful shock rejected the cancer. This effect persisted through a rat's lifetime, long after helplessness or hopefulness was imprinted early in life.

The Depression Connection

Rats, however, are far simpler creatures than human beings. You can't put a human being into a cage and shock him to find out if he's an optimist or a pessimist, or to find out how much of his fatigue is conditioned by his thinking. How, then, can you determine the strength of a person's optimism, and how it might affect his energy levels? Seligman found that the way a person *explains* events to himself is the clue. For example, if a pessimist's spouse walks out of the room, slamming the door, he might think to himself, "My spouse hates me. I'm unlovable." And the optimist might shake his head, shrug and tell himself, "My spouse is in a bad mood. Everybody gets into bad moods sometimes."

Each person has an explanatory style. That style shows how he views the world. According to Seligman, there are three main components to that style:

Stable. An optimist feels life is controllable. When something good happens to him, he feels it is due to his own efforts. When something bad happens, he regards it as a fluke, and still believes he has control over his life. A pessimist feels life is out of his control. If something good happens to him he regards it as a lucky break that probably won't happen again. If something bad happens, it's just proof of the harshness of fate.

Global. The optimist takes good events as proof that all of life is basically good. The pessimist cannot generalize about good events. With a bad event, however, the tables turn dramatically. Optimists refuse to let a bad event "spread," while pessimists let bad events cast a dark, depressing shadow over their entire life.

Internal. Optimists shrug off the bad and internalize the good. "I got a lucky break because I'm a good guy," says the optimist. Pessimists attribute the good to outside forces, and the bad to themselves. "I lost that job because I'm incompetent. I got sick because my immune system is weak."

Optimism penetrates every aspect of a person's life, including his or her health. Optimists tend to believe they have control over their health, and so they are more likely to exercise, seek medical advice, and follow a healthful lifestyle. One study has shown the remarkable impact of hope on health by following two hundred exceptionally gifted and physically fit men at Harvard for the last fifty years. Psychoanalyst George Vaillant, who has directed the study, has found that optimists are far healthier and more energetic in middle and old age than their pessimistic counterparts. Even when Seligman analyzed the sports-page quotes of thirty-four Baseball Hall of Famers who played between 1900 and 1950, pessimists—who thought their triumphs were due to "luck"—lived significantly shorter lives than inveterate optimists.

So, what do you do if you feel you are a "born" pessimist? The good news is that explanatory style can be changed. The tool is cognitive therapy, in which the therapist and patient examine—and alter—pessimist thought patterns. This therapy can often be fairly short-term (a matter of weeks or months). Studies have shown that this type of therapy is as successful as drugs in treating depression.

Doctors of all kinds are now coming to recognize the impact of stress on the body. Studies have shown that job stress can actually be linked to *structural* changes in the heart that make an individual more susceptible to heart disease. Changing your response to stress is a first step to dismantling chronic fatigue, and it's a subject we'll look at in depth later on in this book.

As Martin Seligman points out, "Life inflicts the same setbacks and tragedies on the optimist as on the pessimist, but the optimist weathers them better."

When you catch yourself connecting adversity with beliefs that lead to depression, you can use several tactics:

Use Seligman's methods of distraction (start an activity, whether it's taking a walk in the woods, calling a friend, watching a movie, exercising) and disputation (arguing with yourself). The latter can be extremely effective. Your first argument with yourself might be as follows, "I feel sick and tired, and I feel as though I'm never going to get better. But I'm reading Dr. Hoffman's book, and he keeps writing about patients of his who got better. If they got better, so can I."

Another method I recommend to patients is letting their troubles float away. This may sound simplistic, but I've seen it work. Sit in a comfortable chair or lie back on your bed, and imagine your troubles as balloons. Give each balloon the name of a trouble and then simply let it go and watch it float away into a clear blue sky until it simply disappears.

For further, detailed prescriptions on exactly how to change your thinking patterns, consult Dr. Seligman's best-selling book.

The Depression Connection

There are many other techniques for improving your mood and helping combat depression, among them:

1. Address yourself to only one or two problems at a time. Trying to conquer every problem in your life is impossible—and will only leave you feeling helpless and more depressed and tired.

2. Since depression is often associated with sleeplessness, tension, and fatigue, practice relaxation techniques at least once a day. Relaxation has a widespread and beneficial effect on the body. Herbert Benson has written a fine book on the subject, entitled *The Relaxation Response*. Benson became famous after publishing this book, which adapted Eastern meditation techniques to the typical harried American.

To relax, pick a quiet, comfortable spot with few distractions. Try to choose a time at least two hours after a meal, so you won't be sleepy from the digestive process. Then do one of the following:

• Repeat a word silently or aloud, allowing yourself to simply focus on the word.

• Breathe deeply and fully, and observe your breath. Focus your attention on your breath and let all worldly distractions fall from your mind.

• Imagine a peaceful scene, such as a starry night or a warm ocean shore. Imagine the warm sun beating down. Or imagine yourself snuggling under a warm, clean down comforter in a ski resort after exercising all day. Visualize any scene that makes you feel relaxed and safe.

• Let yourself flow into the relaxation.

Don't be surprised if you experience occasional muscle spasms or jerks while you relax, or tingling sensations in your muscles. Don't let them alarm you—these are common responses and are actually signals that you are relaxing.

Once you have mastered the technique of relaxing, use it in situations where you are upset. Hold onto the feeling.

3. Read a self-help book. Authors I like who have written inspiring books include Joan Borysenko, Louise Hay, and Deepak Chopra. Aaron Beck, a father of cognitive therapy, has written several helpful books on changing thinking patterns.

4. Make a list of activities you find pleasant—whether exercising, eating a good meal with friends, accomplishing a task at work, relaxing in a hot bath, or taking a walk in the country. Note down in the course of a week how often you perform those activities. You may be surprised at how little time you allot for pleasurable activities. Now make a schedule where you spend at least thirty minutes a day on activities that make you feel good.

5. If you start to lose yourself in a cascade of negative thinking (I'll never be happy, I'll always be alone, I'll always feel tired), snap a rubber band that you wear around your wrist. This is a technique popular among cognitive therapists—therapists who believe that if you change thinking patterns, you can change your mood. If you are in public when negative thinking occurs, imagine yourself yelling, "STOP!"

The opposite technique sometimes works as well. Blow your negative thoughts out of proportion. Make them even more negative than before. Suppose you're so tired you make a mistake at work, and you're worried that your boss will be furious. Imagine your boss becoming so upset that he or she starts screaming at you hysterically, throws every object in the office against the wall, tears up paper on his desk, and summons every co-worker to hear him loudly pronounce you incompetent.

Let your imagination run amok. Imagining a scene so terrible accomplishes two things: it gives your worst fears an outlet, and at the same time, it appears so ridiculous it's funny. Also, by that time the mere idea that the boss might be upset will seem survivable.

6. Start an exercise program. Researchers believe that strenuous exercise triggers chemical changes in the body that are similar to those caused by antidepressant medications. For one thing, the body's endorphins—our internal, feel-good chemicals—are increased by exercise. But other brain chemicals may be affected as well. Exercise can be an important part of any treatment program for depression.

7. Since depression is sometimes a form of anger turned inward—especially in women, who are socialized to hold in their anger—assertiveness training can be a big help. There are numerous self-help books on becoming assertive. I often recommend that my patients try being assertive for a day. If they feel better, they have a clue to the cause of their depression. There have been times in my life when I

felt I was being too nice and accommodating, and I noticed I was feeling weighted down, depressed, and lethargic. Getting angry in a constructive way can help boost your mood and energy.

8. Imagine yourself as the client of a counselor or therapist who treats psychotics and criminal parolees. Visualize yourself standing in front of yourself. You'll probably find you've been your own worst critic. You'll find that your "counselor's" advice to you is probably more compassionate than you expected. See yourself through the eyes of this sympathetic counselor. Remember that you're human—like everybody else.

9. Try to reframe your approach to your fatigue. For people who have suffered from bona fide chronic fatigue and illness, each new ache and pain is perceived as part of the fabric of illness—reinforcing a doom-and-gloom mentality. As I sit writing these lines my scalp itches, my neck feels tight, and I am experiencing mild bloating after a hearty dinner of vegetarian chili. But I don't weave these fleeting symptoms into a continuing pattern of chronic, all-pervasive illness. I find my chronic fatigue patients, even after they start getting well, are so afraid of remaining sick that every fluctuation in well-being seems a sign of relapse. They wake up every morning and take an inventory: "I'm dizzy again. I'm tired again. I'm sore again." This defeatist attitude is natural and understandable, since for months or years they have been hurting. Cognitive reframing can help them examine symptoms one at a time, and on an individual basis.

Your Energy Plan

Take the depression quiz in this chapter, and if you answer yes to many or most of the questions, consider the possibility that masked depression is contributing to your fatigue.

Change your diet to eliminate refined sugars, caffeine, and chocolate, which may contribute to mood swings.

Emphasize antidepression nutrients, including L-tyrosine, L-phenylalanine, vitamins B6 and B12, magnesium, and vitamin C.

Read self-help books on cognitive reframing.

If your malaise persists, see a health professional.

13

CHRONIC FATIGUE SYNDROME: THE TWENTIETH-CENTURY PLAGUE?

▼

When did chronic fatigue immune dysfunction syndrome become a "real disease"? Perhaps when it was canonized in a cover story in *Newsweek*. Subtitled "A Modern Medical Mystery," this noteworthy article began with the tale of Nancy Kaiser, a woman who in 1974 "made the mistake of coming down with an illness that didn't fit any of the available diagnoses. The Albuquerque housewife was just 38, an avid golfer and swimmer under no particular stress. Yet she felt like she was dying. She was weak, profoundly tired, and plagued by constant bladder infections. Her muscles ached. Her mood shifted unpredictably. Her memory seemed to be failing." Persuaded that certain of her symptoms were hormonal, she agreed to a hysterectomy.

Her health still didn't improve, so she was sent to a psychiatrist, who told her she was mourning her lost uterus. By 1987, Nancy Kaiser had seen 212 different experts. She was having a dozen minor epileptic seizures a day and often lacked the strength to stand up. Finally she found an expert who was willing to help her, and relief came in the form of an antiviral drug, Ampligen. According to the article, she now leads a nearly normal life. And I sat next to her at a CFS conference, chatted with her, and heard her deliver a moving address. If there's hope for "hard-core" patients like Nancy, anyone can find the comeback trail.

Nancy is not that unusual: I see patients like her frequently. Perhaps the most frustrating and rewarding aspect of my practice in the last few years has been the diagnosis and treatment of CFS, since it is a disorder with no clear cause and with debilitating symptoms that can last for years. The toll it takes can be terrible. As Mark Iverson, the president of a CFS association, has said, "I've never known a single person with full-blown CFS who has not considered taking their own life." And if CFS is hard on adults, it's disastrous for children, because it often affects the brain, and children may lose key developmental milestones.

The good news? CFS is not a fatal disease. And eventually, many people begin to recover. Even the sickest patients, like Nancy Kaiser, may suffer for years and then finally find an approach that helps. The path to recovery may be circuitous and long, but many patients find it.

Long before the Centers for Disease Control (CDC) acknowledged this illness as a national epidemic, I was seeing patients who were suffering from what sounded like a bad flu—except they just didn't get better. They suffered from sore throats, swollen lymph glands, low-grade fevers, muscle and joint pain, headaches, and problems with concentration. Exercise made them feel worse, not better. Most of all, the hallmark of their illness seemed to be profound fatigue.

That's why I'm excited by the new national awareness of CFS. Every month, the Centers for Disease Control in Atlanta receives 2,000 calls inquiring about CFS. People at the CDC are now believers—and they are seeing and charting the path of a growing epidemic in this country. It is on the map, and it is real. It's now estimated that 1–2 million Americans have some form of this disorder. An astounding hundred billion dollars in productivity is lost each year as a result of this pervasive syndrome, which can cause long-term disability.

Although nearly 60 percent of my patients come to me with fatigue, only about 10 percent actually have what I would characterize as full-blown CFS. Nonetheless, that is a significant chunk of my practice, and one that leaves indelible images in my mind: I've had patients come in too tired to sit up in a chair; they have recounted their history from an examination table, propped up on pillows.

Because there is no specific test to "prove" you have the syndrome, it is diagnosed by symptoms (usually an array of unexplained symptoms like those of Nancy Kaiser) that severely restrict normal activity and are not due to other diseases of the immune system such as AIDS, cancer, and lupus. These are the typical symptoms of the disease, according to the CDC. I don't follow them strictly, but they are a good guideline:

1. Fatigue for at least six months, usually of rapid onset
2. Mild fever or chills
3. Sore throat
4. Painful lymph nodes in the neck
5. Unexplained muscle weakness
6. Muscle pain
7. Fatigue that lasts twenty-four hours or longer after exercising
8. Headaches
9. Joint pain without swelling or redness
10. Short-term memory problems, forgetfulness, inability to concentrate, occasional difficulty focusing
11. Depression
12. Sleep disturbance—insomnia, or too much sleep

What causes CFS? Although researchers once thought that the Epstein-Barr virus, which causes mononucleosis, was responsible for CFS, they now believe that the disease may be due to many viruses working in concert. The bodies of patients with CFS reveal high antibody counts to many viruses, including cytomegalovirus and members of the herpes family of viruses. And even healthy, asymptomatic family members of a CFS victim have certain immunological abnormalities that suggest the presence of a virus.

Recently, scientists at the Wistar Institute, in Philadelphia, reported a link between a specific virus and chronic fatigue. The virus—a retrovirus—was discovered in several small groups of patients suffering from chronic fatigue, including children in an upstate New York town where an epidemic occurred. The virus was detected through extremely sophisticated laboratory tests. Though the discovery does not prove that chronic fatigue is caused by a single specific virus, it supports the increasingly popular theory that many of our chronic diseases may implicate viruses.

According to Paul Cheney, one of the pioneering physicians in this epidemic, over half of all CFS patients reported a domestic pet that suffered a serious illness or died. There also seems to be a higher incidence of cancer in close relatives of people with CFS. In one study, 35 patients reported 38 cancers in first-order relatives (siblings, parents, children). There's a lot of cancer in this country, but 38 cancers in 205 first-order relatives is alarming. The link might be a genetic factor, as well as a virus.

CFS may actually have its origins in an old disorder. It resembles diseases described in the late nineteenth and early twentieth century, such as neurasthenia (exhaustion and listlessness), and an illness known as myalgic encephalomyelitis, or ME, which has been described in medical reports for at least half a century.

A third disorder, called fibrositis or fibromyalgia, was first described in the nineteenth century, and it has many striking similarities to CFS. Soft-tissue pain, particularly tender points along various muscles, is a hallmark of fibromyalgia, though fatigue, sore throats, and other aches and pains are also prominent symptoms. Fibromyalgia occurs predominantly in women (80 percent of patients) of childbearing age. It sounds like some cases of CFS, but it is not: Pain control in this disease is especially enhanced by exercise and stretching, which relieves muscle pain and achiness. In CFS patients, exercise intensifies the illness. Nonetheless, fibromyalgia patients demonstrate certain immune-system abnormalities, along with sleep disorders, and can be helped by many of the same treatments that help CFS sufferers.

The new theory is that CFS begins when a toxic agent (either a potent virus, a chemical toxin, or perhaps another microbe, such as pathogenic yeast) damages the immune system. Other latent viruses usually held in check then start reproducing rapidly. These include viruses in the herpes family (Epstein-Barr, cytomegalovirus, herpes simplex 1 and 2, and human herpes virus 6) and enteroviruses (Coxsackie virus and echovirus). Most of these viruses infect us in our childhood, and our bodies learn to keep them in check. Ninety percent of human beings have at least one herpes family virus in their body.

When CFS strikes, the immune system goes on red alert, and certain immune-system cells (known as suppressor T-cells) often become overactivated. This can exacerbate allergies, which further weaken the immune system. The body wages a losing war in fighting all of these attacks, and laboratory tests have found that the "natural killer" cells of patients with this disorder are extremely sluggish in the test tube.

Chronic Fatigue Syndrome: The Twentieth-Century Plague?

One reason CFS patients may feel so sick is that their immune systems, fighting desperately, release a lot of cytokines, which are chemicals that do battle against foreign invaders. These chemicals—called interleukin-1, interleukin-2, and interferon—are responsible for many of the flulike symptoms you feel whenever you are sick. Even cancer patients given these immune boosters end up with flulike malaise and fatigue. We can test CFS patients for the levels of these cytokines; their presence is a clue to the presence of the disease.

Although CFS has been nicknamed the "yuppie flu," it strikes all ages and doesn't discriminate between class, gender, and race. In Incline Village, Nevada, it struck nearly two hundred residents.

Until recently, many physicians believed CFS was a variant of depression or perhaps hypochondria. But a major study by physicians Andrew Lloyd and Dennis Wakefield investigated forty-eight CFS patients and found that depression was a consequence, not a cause, of the illness. Recurrent sore throats, swollen glands, and low-grade fevers are not the clinical picture of depression or anxiety. In addition, studies at Mount Sinai Hospital in New York, by physician Susan Levine, have found that CFS patients make more norepinephrine, better known as adrenaline. The longer they've been sick, the more adrenaline they put out. That means they may suffer from anxiety and panic disorders as a *result* of the stress of their disease. One way to tell if patients have genuine, primary panic disorder is to give them sedatives. If they have primary panic disorder, they will feel better. If they're suffering from CFS, they will usually feel even sicker.

CFS leads to specific changes in a patient's memory and ability to perform tasks. CFS can and often does damage the nervous system, which is why, when people say, "It's all in your head," they are actually telling a certain kind of truth. I have a CFS patient who was a systems analyst for a big company. On her first visit to my office I asked her to count backward from 100 by seven (100, 93, 86, 79, 72 . . .), which is called the serial seven subtraction test. It's a standard test for evaluating people for premature senility, and not extremely difficult, but she was completely thrown by it. Clinically, this test is a pearl, because so many patients with CFS just can't do it readily. They can't even balance their checkbooks.

How does a doctor diagnose CFS? It's hard to prove—yet easy to spot simply by the constellation of symptoms. As far as lab tests go, however, CFS is elusive and tricky. Some patients with CFS end up with false positives on blood tests for lupus. That's because they have a similar autoimmune glitch in their system—but it doesn't mean they have lupus, and a misdiagnosis can cause untold emotional turmoil. Similarly, I've seen patients with too many suppressor T-cells, and others with too many helper T-cells (a signal that the immune system is in an alarm state). In Japan, where they call CFS "Natural Killer Cell Disease," they claim that patients have almost no natural killer cells in their immune system. I've seen that situation, but I've also seen rare CFS patients with an overproliferation of natural killer cells.

A new test—for something called the angiotensin-converting enzyme—is positive in many CFS cases, but also in Lyme disease. Lyme disease is caused by a spirochete, a tiny microbe transmitted by ticks. Since the ticks are extremely small (smaller than a pinhead), the bites often painless, and the initial symptoms vague, the disease can sometimes go undiagnosed for years while sufferers succumb to a wide range of symptoms such as debilitating fatigue, joint problems, neurological difficulties, and susceptibility to other infections. Lyme disease can be hard to diagnose, because the test generally available for the disease is an antibody test, rather than a test for the spirochete itself. Some immune-compromised individuals may not manufacture enough antibodies to result in a positive test, while other individuals may have antibodies to syphilis, another spirochete, which may cross-react with the Lyme test and cause a false positive. To ensure the highest possible accuracy for the test, I recommend testing at a university laboratory that is skilled in this area. For those on the East Coast, the State University of New York at Stony Brook on Long Island is renowned for pioneering work in Lyme disease. A special department at Yale University Medical School, another top Lyme disease center, recently announced plans to develop a Lyme vaccine.

When I get a patient with a positive test for Lyme, or a negative test associated with puzzling symptoms that began after a camping trip in a tick-infested area, I experience a dilemma: Do I give them major doses of antibiotics to kill a Lyme disease microbe that they may not actually have? Unnecessary antibiotics may strike a serious blow to their immune system. On the other hand, untreated Lyme can result in dire complications, such as arthritis and nerve damage. I make the final decision individually, case by case.

The truth about CFS, as I see it at this writing, is that there are many different patterns of the disease. I've seen CFS patients whose symptoms consist primarily of bladder problems, others who suffer from aches and malaise, still others who suffer from constant muscular twitching and muscle pain. Each person's body may express the disease differently, but all the patients have one thing in common: their immune system is dysregulated, causing constant malaise and illness.

Beware of physicians who test you for Epstein-Barr or cytomegalovirus, then dismiss you. This is a tack I've seen many conventional physicians take now that they're aware of CFS. The patient comes in, exhausted; the physician takes tests for these two viruses, and almost inevitably finds elevated "titers" (or levels of antibodies). The doctor pronounces the patient infected with one or both of these viruses. The condition now has a "name." But the truth is, these are antibodies to ubiquitous viruses that are often present at high levels in healthy individuals. The titers don't help us define the disease. I haven't used such tests in several years and feel they're generally a waste of money. New molecular probes for traces of active, replicating virus, called PCR tests, may eventually supplant the old antibody tests.

To me, this "find-a-bug" approach is ultimately bankrupt. CFS is probably due to a mysterious and highly individual mélange of viruses, yeasts, allergies, chemical and heavy-metal poisons, and stress. Hormones may also play a role, since pregnancy reduces the effects of CFS, just as it reduces the severity of autoimmune diseases like multiple sclerosis. (During pregnancy, high levels of progesterone help create immune tolerance to prevent miscarriage.)

My first approach to CFS is to rule out other causes of illness—not just lupus or Lyme disease, but multiple chemical sensitivity, mold allergies, or sleep disorders, all of which can masquerade as CFS. What a relief to such patients when they are freed of the lifelong sentence of CFS!

You can't "prove" the existence of CFS, but you can run some extremely sensitive tests that pick up abnormalities in the immune system. These tests, along with a symptom history, can usually pinpoint the presence of CFS. Here are some that I use:

Tests for levels of natural killer cells—immune system warriors.

Tests for changed levels of immune proteins called immune globulins: IgG, subsets 1 through 4, IgA, IgM, IgE. They indicate the presence of chronic infection, allergy, or immune suppression.

Jay Levy, a physician-researcher in San Francisco, has described a particular pattern of immune-system abnormality involving subsets of suppressor T-cells that may actually define genuine chronic fatigue syndrome. I've found it a useful test for differentiating chronic fatigue from other maladies, if performed by several specialized laboratories, including ImmunoDiagnostic Laboratories in San Leandro, California. Tell your doctor to request the Suppressor T-Cell Subset panel.

In addition, molecular assay for a by-product of viral replication, 2-5-A synthetase, is a sensitive measure of viral activity but does not distinguish among viruses.

CFS is treatable. Yet the range of treatments stretches from here to eternity. It is important to offer patients two things:

Believe what they are saying—that they are suffering real symptoms of a real disease.

Give treatments that have demonstrated significant, tangible improvement in a substantial number of sufferers. What CFS patients fear the most is that they will go on suffering . . . and suffering . . . and suffering. As one reporter and CFS victim, Hillary Johnson, reported in an article, "I couldn't bear to talk to people who had been sick longer than I had . . . it was too threatening, and it was one reason I had little interest in joining a support group."

I've found that each CFS patient is highly individual and may respond magnificently to a treatment that doesn't help another individual at all. We just keep trying to boost the immune system, and allow it to recover slowly. And, over time, it usually does. A typical CFS patient of mine was a healthy, burn-the-candle-at-both-ends woman of twenty-eight who came down with mononucleosis and, as so many of these patients tell me, "never got better." Even so, she went back to work after six weeks, but she grew increasingly worse over the next year, until all she could do was drag herself to the office and drag herself home. She became completely isolated from her friends because she never had the energy to see them. Finally she quit her job and moved in with her mother. I treated her with weekly intravenous vitamin C—at doses of forty grams—along with allergy shots, candida treatment, and a rotating diet. A year later she was substantially improved, had gone back to work part-time, and had resumed her daily swimming. Nonetheless, she was still dependent on the vitamin C drips and still vulnerable to infection: when she came down with strep throat it took her three weeks to recover (it usually takes about ten days), and it caused a flare-up in her CFS symptoms.

Until recently, the most common treatment offered to CFS patients was antidepressant medication. Although some sufferers claim that low doses of antidepressants are helpful, I generally try to avoid this approach. Some doctors claim that CFS patients using low-dose Prozac have improved tremendously. I just don't find this in my practice. My CFS patients are so debilitated that they have to be extraordinarily careful about dosages of any and all drugs: they need extremely low amounts. I've found that antidepressants further challenge their fragile immune systems, giving the liver one more chemical to detoxify. One of my patients claims taking these drugs is like the old joke about an alcoholic: "Give a drunk coffee, and you end up with a wide-awake drunk."

Perhaps the simplest, safest "low-tech" approach is intravenous vitamin C. Vitamin C is of enormous importance in the function of the immune system, and when offered intravenously it bypasses the digestive system (which may be faulty), going directly to the cells where it is needed. In addition, I prescribe a new form of oral vitamin C, called "Ester C," which is a complex mixture of many forms of vitamin C, along with minerals that increase its absorption. In a study by Meridian Valley Clinical Laboratories, twelve men aged twenty-seven to forty-five were studied, and it was found that Ester C produced significantly higher concentrations of the vitamin in the blood and white blood cells as long as twenty-four hours later. Far less vitamin C was excreted in the urine.

Studies show that vitamin C stimulates the production of white blood cells, inactivates a variety of viruses and bacteria in test tubes, shortens the duration of colds, and reduces the symptoms of asthma and allergies. Vitamin C is needed by the adrenal glands to synthesize hormones, and though these glands normally contain high levels of vitamin C, they are depleted during stress. Some CFS patients have shown only 20 percent of normal levels of ascorbic acid.

Though vitamin C has many potential benefits, human beings are at high risk for deficiencies of the vitamin. All other mammals produce their own vitamin C. Primates and guinea pigs eat the equivalent of 10,000 milligrams of vitamin C a day when under stress. Even the caveman diet of centuries ago contained about 400 milligrams of vitamin C daily, and yet the current RDA is only 60 milligrams.

There are conflicting studies about the role of vitamin C in treating cancer. Because it boosts the immune system, some doctors prescribe the vitamin along with traditional chemotherapy. In one study, 10 grams of vitamin C were given daily to "hopelessly ill" cancer patients. They survived about three hundred days longer than control subjects. And one out of five survived over a year longer than expected, compared with only 0.4 percent of controls. However, other studies have not shown such positive results. Whether or not the vitamin can help treat cancer, it certainly can help prevent it—and cancer may be a concern for CFS patients, because, as I mentioned earlier, anecdotal evidence indicates their risk may be higher. The National Cancer Institute recommends a diet high in the vitamin, and a recent NCI symposium revealed that of 46 studies on the effects of vitamin C in human cancer, 33 showed statistically significant protection. The studies dealt with everything from oral cancer to stomach, pancreas, cervical, rectal, colon, and breast cancer.

Vitamin C *is* found in high amounts in broccoli, brussels sprouts, black currants, kale, sweet peppers, lemon pulp, orange pulp, mustard greens, strawberries, and watercress. Moderate sources of the vitamin include grapefruit, limes, melons, potatoes, turnips, tangerines, asparagus, and lima beans.

There is no proven toxicity for vitamin C. Some studies once suggested it might cause kidney stones, but subsequent studies have shown there is no such link in normal, healthy people. For those with kidney disease, high doses of vitamin C may cause a problem. Other studies suggested that taking high doses of vitamin C and suddenly stopping may induce a kind of "rebound scurvy." A recent study found no basis for this suggestion.

I also include other, synergistic nutrients in vitamin C infusions, including zinc, which stimulates immunity and directly inhibits the common cold virus; vitamin B6, which stimulates antibody response and supports the adrenal glands; and vitamin B5, which is a building block for cortisone and strengthens the adrenal glands.

Other herbs and nutritional supplements can help boost the immune system, including extracts of shiitake and reishi mushrooms, which have been shown to have immune-stimulating properties; garlic, which is antibacterial and can stimulate the NK (natural killer) cells of the immune system; coenzyme Q-10, also known as ubiquinone, which is extremely important for all energy reactions in cells; dimethyl glycine, or DMG, which stimulates oxygen uptake and cellular immunity; Ginkgo biloba, a venerable ancient herb that has been proved to stimulate circulation and improve memory and concentration; and antioxidants like glutathione, which are important for liver detoxification.

Magnesium is another hugely important nutrient, which can be given intravenously or orally. A study reported in the prestigious British journal *The Lancet,* in March of 1991, found that magnesium given by injection is of considerable benefit to patients with CFS, particularly those with muscle aches. Twenty patients had the magnesium in their red blood cells measured and then compared with that of twenty healthy subjects. The CFS patients showed significantly lower red-cell magnesium levels. Then thirty-five CFS patients with proven low magnesium levels were given either a placebo or magnesium injections for six weeks. The patients on magnesium were substantially improved. Magnesium helps reduce anxiety, as well.

For more information about nutritional supplements, consult *The Real Vitamin and Mineral Book,* by Shari Lieberman and Nancy Bruning (Avery Publishing Group, 1990). You can find this book in many health-food stores and in health-oriented sections of regular bookstores.

There may be another potent new treatment for CFS. The drug, called Kutapressin, is a liver extract that was originally developed in the late 1940s and has been used for years to control inflammations of the skin ranging from adult acne to poison ivy. Though physicians are not sure exactly how it works, it seems to help reduce inflammation at the cellular level. Kutapressin is administered by injection into the muscle of the buttocks and is considered extremely safe.

In 1983, doctors at Memorial City Medical Center in Houston began using Kutapressin to treat chronic fatigue in 270 patients. The doctors hypothesized that chronic fatigue was the result of an immune system that was out of balance—triggered by viral infections, severe allergic reactions, stress, or other toxins. The immune system doesn't recover fully from these stresses, begins to overreact to all kinds of stimuli, and is soon exhausted. Since Kutapressin has been shown to help reduce herpes outbreaks, it was tried on patients with chronic fatigue. Patients had been suffering for at least four months and were given tests to determine immune dysregulation, as well as tests to rule out other illnesses, like Lyme disease or lupus. The drug was injected every day for four to ten days and then every other day until patients recovered.

The astounding good news: 95 percent of patients improved significantly, although some required as many as eighty or ninety injections. Most patients required about thirty to forty. Most of the patients in the study had had symptoms for more than a year, and had received treatments ranging from vitamins to drugs, gamma globulin, antidepressants, and antihistamines. Almost none of the patients had improved. According to the research, "the majority of patients began their improvement after the tenth injection." Progress occurred in plateaus—suddenly the patient would feel better and then would plateau for a while before experiencing another leap in well-being. When patients suffered from minor setbacks, such as a flu or sudden stress, they returned to daily injections for a week or two until they felt better again.

Some doctors recommend injections of gamma globulin. Gamma globulin is a fraction of the blood that contains antibodies. You may be familiar with it if you've traveled to tropical regions and your doctor has recommended a booster to protect you against hepatitis and other infections. Some CFS patients have improved with high doses of intravenous gamma globulin, but I recommend it only rarely, when the immune system is so obviously depressed that insurance companies will cover the exorbitant cost: as we have noted earlier, a single infusion can cost up to a thousand dollars, and the average patient needs one every several weeks for many months. Gamma globulin is generally well tolerated, and the risk of acquiring hepatitis or HIV is thought to be negligible, thanks to improved methods of screening and sterilization.

Transfer factor is another extract, with over one hundred peptides taken from the white blood cells of healthy individuals. Transfer factor can stimulate all facets of the immune response, and so it must be administered carefully, as it can increase some of the T-cells that are responsible for autoimmune and allergic reactions. Its availability is limited and it, too, is costly.

Other new therapies that can be helpful include:

1. Ampligen, an antiviral drug that helped Nancy Kaiser, whose story is told at the beginning of this chapter. It is currently being delayed for approval by the FDA.

2. Homeopathic doses of Cortrosyn—a form of ACTH, which is an adrenal hormone. When this is titrated to millionth-of-a-gram doses, it can have a gentle, homeostatic effect on exhausted adrenal glands.

3. Extremely small doses of a flu vaccine called Fluogen, along with very dilute doses of rubella vaccine. Even though the flu and rubella viruses are different from Epstein-Barr and other typical viruses that are activated during CFS, a very mild, dilute dose of flu and rubella can induce a tiny immune response that subtly regulates an overstimulated nervous system.

Studies show that some chronic fatigue patients have improved using these therapies. The doses have to be very carefully administered—the treatment is similar to provocation/neutralization used for allergies—by a physician skilled in environmental medicine.

For more information, order *CFIDS: An Owner's Manual,* by Barbara Brooke and Nancy Smith, with Andrew N. Guthrie (BBNS Publishers, Silver Spring, Maryland). Also good is *Solving the Puzzle of Chronic Fatigue Syndrome,* by Michael Rosenbaum and Murray Susser (Life Sciences Press, Tacoma), and *Chronic Fatigue Syndrome* and *The Yeast Connection,* by William G. Crook, M.D.

Your Energy Plan

Contact the national CFIDS Association at P.O. Box 220398, Charlotte, North Carolina 28222-0398, for a list of doctors specializing in this illness. Or write to Jay Goldstein, M.D., editor of *Journal of the Chronic Fatigue Syndromes,* 500 S. Anaheim Hills Road, Suite 128, Anaheim Hills, California 92807, for a sample copy of a new journal detailing the latest innovative drugs and treatments for CFS from around the world.

Tired All the Time

Ask a CFS specialist to give you the latest, most sensitive tests to spot immune abnormalities associated with CFS.

Join a CFS support group.

Try some of the newest treatments for chronic viral infections, including:

Intravenous vitamin C infusions

Magnesium injections

Injections of Kutapressin, a liver peptide

In rare cases, transfer factor and gamma globulin

Immune-boosting herbs such as echinacea, and minerals such as zinc

Extremely low-dose dilutions of flu and rubella vaccines

Homeopathic low doses of Cortrosyn, an adrenal hormone

14

SURVIVING SUCCESS: MAINTAINING HIGH ENERGY LEVELS

▼

Why is the Buddha fat and smiling?

The weight of the world is upon him, the supreme question of good and evil seems to hang in daily balance, and his tens of thousands of followers plague him hourly, but he simply sits calmly throughout eternity, an enigmatic smile upon his lips. I tell my patients he is smiling because he has learned the art of handling stress: he doesn't let much in this world upset him.

Sometimes nothing is wrong with an exhausted person—except the fact that he or she has been racing like Road Runner for the last ten years, packing in every possible experience without the time to stop and savor life.

One of the most memorable men I ever met was a neurosurgeon in his sixties—and he had the Buddha's gift of tirelessness. I was a young resident physician in his hospital, and I watched him work from about 7 A.M. until eight or nine at night. He performed excruciatingly delicate operations for hours a day and handled enormous teaching responsibilities. I rarely saw him eat, and when he did, it was a tiny sandwich on white bread. It seemed as if his response to stress was to calm down. He was like one of those economy cars that get rated at 62 miles per gallon—not only because of fuel efficiency but also because their test drivers slow down long before a stoplight and accelerate very gently. He did everything with an astonishing, perfect parsimony of effort, and even his gestures and voice seemed calibrated. He was the consummate doctor.

I see patients in my practice every day who are as active and successful as that neurosurgeon—but many of them are also breaking down under the crushing weight of stress in their lives. They suffer from exhaustion, physical ills, and emotional fragility. Perhaps because I live in Manhattan, a city of ambitious high achievers, I see more of these workaholics than some other doctors. And I secretly sympathize with them, because they're people after my own heart. I, too, find it hard to slow down. Whenever I leave New York, I feel tremendously depressurized—and I start to miss the self-contained madness of the city. I have an affinity for New York and for my patients who are stressed. Stress can move you to excellence and provide an opportunity for great productivity. I almost never take a vacation, and my schedule is so hectic that I haven't yet had time to move out of the cramped, fifth-floor apartment I've lived in for the last two decades. But I *have* learned to moderate my internal clock—to pause, to rest, to laugh. Why achieve success if you can't survive it?

For many of us, achieving success is not the hardest task in life. Staying aloft—and negotiating stress—is the real art. Life will always generate stress, and as you get older, difficulties accumulate. Maintaining longevity and health isn't easy or automatic. There are four basic ways to do so, and these energy boosters can help any driven high achiever:

1. Give up addictions, such as caffeine, cigarettes, and alcohol, that you believe are helping you "cope" with stress. The truth is that these addictive substances are only short-term palliatives. In the long run, they add to stress.

2. Substitute positive "addictions," such as exercise, creative hobbies, relaxation, and biofeedback. These behaviors will not only balance and calm your system, they will strengthen it.

3. Build up your bulwark against stress. Find out if you have deficiencies of vitamins and minerals, nutrients, enzymes, sleep, or hormones.

4. Reframe your beliefs about the world so that stress won't pack such a wallop. Too many people have the mistaken belief that they should be constantly riding the crest of an "energy high." When we talk about energy, we really need to talk about suppleness of response—the ability to accomplish a task and then slow down and relax. Energy is not like an electric light that you can turn on and leave on until it burns out.

• • • •

Stress is not what it used to be. We are a generation of Americans who impose a huge burden of achievement upon ourselves. We are grade-conscious, time-conscious, score-conscious. An example from the world of athletics is the marathon. As marathon runners know, stress isn't necessarily a bad thing. It can stimulate, strengthen, and challenge you. Exercise, for instance, stresses bone so that your body builds new bone—and therefore helps prevent osteoporosis. And stress can sometimes be like the heat of a kiln, which fires a clay pot so that it won't shatter. It can condition you. Even almost unbearable stress can sometimes force a burst of tremendous creativity—think of the genius of a Dostoevsky, who was so stressed by his gambling debts that he produced some of his later masterworks in a matter of months, dictating around the clock to an eighteen-year-old girl (whom he later married out of gratitude).

Many of us are actually addicted to stress, to the thrill of the challenge and the kick of the stress-related chemicals our body produces. Like Dostoevsky, some of us can't produce unless stress is firing off alarm signals every moment. And some of us can't feel pleasure without stress. At rock concerts we blast our eardrums, at horror movies we succumb to special-effects images and sounds primed to elicit a very visceral stress response. Our palms sweat. Our hearts race. I was reminded of this recently when I saw the famous 3-D Michael Jackson video at the Epcot Center in Disney World. The music was thudding, the images were hypnotic, and Michael Jackson loomed so close you could practically see his nostrils flare. The audience loved it.

One of the first things I ask patients to do is evaluate their own need for stress. Some questions I ask:

• Do you take vacations? If so, are you able to relax and enjoy them? Or are you always phoning the office or bringing work along to do at poolside?

• Are your days packed with appointments? Do you run from work to dinner to an evening with friends or clients?

• Do you thrive on caffeine and other stimulants?

• Do you love the bustle of cities? Does the thought of a small, sleepy town in Iowa sound like purgatory?

• Can you function for a day without a clock or watch? Or does the mere thought of not knowing what time it is make you uneasy?

• Are you one of those people who say, "I know I should meditate, I know I should try yoga, but I just can't be still that long"?

Before you can tackle fatigue, you have to be honest about your taste for stress. Not surprisingly, I find that many chronically exhausted people shudder at the thought of a so-called peaceful, no-stress life.

To love stress is not all bad. Some stress is good. It's simply important to achieve a balance. How do you draw the line between exercise that builds muscles or burns them to exhaustion? Why have ulcers developed overnight in previously healthy people during air raids? What about common childhood illnesses like measles and chicken pox? They're "stressors," and they can hurt you or help you. Some stressors challenge the developing immune system, which then protects against these diseases for life. Other stressors permanently damage the immune and nervous systems.

Two years ago, one of my most acutely stressed patients was Nancy M., a forty-eight-year-old journalist who seemed to have walked out of a film noir into my office. She was divorced and a mother of two, and she was testifying on a grand jury against three leaders of organized crime. She had no idea when or if they might retaliate by making an attempt on her life. She sat down, placed her paper cup of coffee on my desk, smoothed back her curly brown hair, and said in a smoker's rasp, "I have panic attacks—my heart pounds. I have terrible chest pains, feel freezing and then like I'm burning up, and I'm nervous, always nervous." Indeed, her hands were trembling as she spoke.

She had been given a prescription for a common tranquilizer, Xanax, by her doctor, but she complained it didn't help at all. She smoked three packs of cigarettes a day, and when I asked why she couldn't cut down, she said she was too stressed. As she pointed out, "I'm always in personal danger. I'm testifying against men who could have me killed any time."

Nancy M. needed a many-faceted approach to her stressful life, and the first step was to help her quit smoking. I asked her why she smoked, and she instantly answered, "I smoke to relax!" I told her that when a physiological craving is linked to the premise that it reduces stress, it is very hard to break. The addiction takes on a life of its own. In fact, people may unwittingly accentuate their stress to provide a pretext for their addictive behavior. Instead of two or three stressful moments a day, stress may crop up twenty to thirty times a day at convenient twenty-minute intervals. Guilt and loss of self-esteem over the addiction may even add to the stress. I told Nancy that smoking was not reducing her stress, and that in fact when she let go of it, her stress would be lessened. She shook her head.

"I can't quit now, Dr. Hoffman. I'm just overwhelmed."

Many patients give me that circular argument: "I can't alleviate the stress that smoking is causing, because I'm under too much stress!" So I did a test called a Lung Check, which analyzes a sample of sputum. The Lung Check is one of my favorite "motivational" tests, and was recently validated in a major medical journal, where it was shown to be more effective than the traditional X ray in getting smokers to quit. In Nancy's case, the results showed precancerous changes associated with marked irritation of the bronchial mucosa. Like many of my patients, Nancy only had to hear the word cancer and see photographs of her own seared lung cells to give up a habit that had seemed to rule her daily existence for twenty years. As you may recall, this is the first step in my four-pronged approach to stress: Give up unhealthful addictions.

Nancy's chest pains, as much as they frightened her, were not serious and did not indicate heart disease. Testing showed she suffered from mitral valve prolapse—a condition of the heart that is usually benign but associated with an exquisitely tuned nervous system that responds in a lightning flash to stress, leaving a person alternately exhausted and totally hyperactive. When heart specialists listen to the "lub-dub-dub" of that mighty pump, 10–20 percent of healthy women have a murmur caused by an abnormally shaped mitral valve. The condition can be confirmed with a noninvasive test called an echocardiogram. These patients are very prone to phantom chest pains, palpitations, fatigue, dizziness, anxiety, and hyperventilation. When I explained that to Nancy, she relaxed a little.

Another "addiction" Nancy had was a masked allergy to corn. We tested her in our allergy laboratory, and once she eliminated corn from her diet, some of her heart symptoms improved. In addition, we gradually tapered her off tranquilizers. These provided temporary relief of her anxiety symptoms, but when they wore off, Nancy suffered nasty rebound symptoms of agitation.

Rule number two: Substitute "beneficial" addictions. In Nancy's case, this was a program of moderate aerobic exercise three times a week. Consistent aerobic exercise can condition the heart and markedly reduce the symptoms of mitral valve prolapse.

To bolster Nancy's bulwark against stress, I tested her nutritional status, and I found that she was low in B vitamins, vitamin E (this gem of a vitamin helps heal mucosal tissue and neutralize the cancer-causing free radicals produced by cigarette smoking), and magnesium. For the past two years, Nancy has been taking the intravenous vitamin and mineral drip called a "Meyers' cocktail," which contains vitamin C, B vitamins, and magnesium. Magnesium is what I call the stress mineral: it has been shown to be a stabilizer of the heart, to reduce palpitations, to calm irritable bowel syndrome, and to lower blood pressure. That's because it's a smooth muscle relaxer, prevents spasms, cramps and arrhythmias, and is depleted by stress, diarrhea, or a diet high in sugar and processed foods. Nancy says that when she misses her monthly Meyers' cocktail, her stress symptoms begin to reappear.

Even though Nancy has finished testifying, she has admitted to me that she may be in personal danger for the rest of her life. "The danger will never disappear, doctor. After all, I haven't joined a witness-protection program. But I'm coping with stress better than I ever have."

Many times I find that a patient who seems terribly emotionally stressed—and who seems to be a candidate for the analyst's couch—is actually physically depleted. A young woman came into my office recently. "I am so stressed out I'm going to lose my job and my relationship," said Roxanne. "I'm just extremely temperamental. When anyone criticizes me at the office I rush into the bathroom and end up crying hysterically. And I'm so thin-skinned with my boyfriend he's threatening to break off our relationship."

I asked her if her stress seemed cyclical, and she said no. However, when I pursued this line of questioning and asked her about her menstrual cycle, she mentioned that she had severe PMS. "I used to be irritable and emotionally fragile for three days before my period. Now it's two weeks before and one week after. I only have one good week a month. It's hard to know when the PMS leaves off and normalcy begins."

"I have a hunch your stress is linked to PMS and nutritional deficiencies," I told her, and recommended a low-sugar diet, along with five important supplements: evening primrose oil (to boost essential fatty acids that help modulate inflammation), vitamin E, magnesium, B6, and zinc. I told her to come back in six weeks. I believed that Roxanne had been deficient in (or had unusually high, inherited requirements for) these nutrients for years. Each time her menstrual cycle "stressed" her, her body was less able to mount a defense. Eventually she was "stressed" three weeks out of four. An old saying about such borderline malnutrition is that it is like an iceberg, largely hidden until hit by the *Titanic* of stress.

Roxanne didn't return until two months later, and did so only to thank me. "The most remarkable thing has happened with those little supplements," she confessed. "My life is completely different. I can handle stress now."

Roxanne was suffering from a nutritional deficiency that was manifesting as PMS, and resulting in a huge amount of life stress. She had labeled herself hysterical and fragile. In truth, she was neither.

People often ask, "Are there really stress vitamins and nutrients?" The answer is yes, in a limited sense. Though the foes of nutritional supplementation think the idea of stress vitamins is simply marketing hype, nutrition does indeed play a significant role in combating stress. It has been shown that extreme physical stress depletes certain nutrients preferentially. For instance, great stress depletes tyrosine, an amino acid. One of the crueler stress experiments involves rats who are forced to swim until they sink. When rats are given extra tyrosine, their ability to swim is extended. The stress of constant emotional arousal is a drain on magnesium. The stress of infection depletes vitamin C, and when animals are under stress they produce as much as sixty times their normal amount of vitamin C. Humans and guinea pigs are the only animals who don't manufacture their own vitamin C, and so supplementation during times of stress can be beneficial.

At the beginning of this chapter, I talked about the fact that some of us are hooked on stress and can't bear to relinquish it. We may be tired, but we're wired at the same time, and we can't seem to slow down. There's a trick to rechanneling the energy of a stress junkie. It does no good to ask a stress lover to sit down and relax, much less meditate. A whole generation of Americans trekked through Nepal to sit in dank caves with their legs painfully crossed awaiting the moment when enlightenment would still their chattering internal monologue. Some of them found it, and Herbert Benson of Harvard University revolutionized the modern approach to meditation when he called it "the Relaxation Response" and proved with laboratory tests that it was enormously beneficial to the body. But many of those individuals waited in vain, and there are many more who are so keyed up they can't stay in one place long enough to relax. And maybe they shouldn't. Relaxation cannot be willed, waited for, or chanted into existence. It's a physiological response.

For patients who would benefit enormously from relaxation but who refuse to pause in mid-flight to try it, a program of exercise can be a miracle worker. Recovering from exertion, the nervous system can begin to access true physiological relaxation.

I often tell my patients that the key to their health and lives is ultimately not simply achieving success. Many of my patients are quite successful in their various walks of life. Their success, however, is a built-in time bomb that eventually impacts their health, depletes their energy, and subjects them to chronic illness. The hallmark of true success is surviving success—and flourishing.

For too many patients, success becomes an addiction, something to be achieved at all costs, leading to physical deterioration, weakness, and breakdown. I think of the joke sometimes seen on bumper stickers: "He who has the most toys at the end of the game wins." That ethos is not a healthy or balanced one. Some physicians theorize the overdrive for success is one cause for the higher incidence of full-blown CFS among so-called yuppies, with the disparaging label "yuppie flu."

Unfortunately, fatigue has become a byword of our existence. Achieving balance is what life is all about, and this book should help you not only design your fatigue wheel and pinpoint your liabilities but also design a health wheel, one that contains a balanced diet, exercise, relaxation, quality sleep. For each exhausting "problem," whether it's allergies or endocrine problems or depression, make a pie slice that embodies a medical or self-care solution.

There's a truism often quoted among environmental physicians: When you're sitting on five tacks, and you remove one of them, how

TIT FOR TAT—THE STRESSLESS WAY TO SUCCESS

▼

Birds do it. Bees do it. So do microbes, primates, married couples, companies, and superpowers. Cooperate, that is. Cooperation often triumphs over fierce competition, according to Robert Axelrod, a professor of political science and public policy at the University of Michigan in Ann Arbor. And cooperation is certainly a low-stress way to achieve what you want.

Axelrod first got on the trail of cooperation while analyzing war. He knew from accounts of World War I that periods of days and weeks elapsed during which neither enemy attacked the other. Axelrod eventually found the answer to their peacekeeping in a game called the Prisoner's Dilemma, which mimics real-life choices in the trenches. The game was invented in 1950 by researchers and has fascinated sociologists for years. It takes two players, who engage in an ongoing contest. Their choices are either to "cooperate" with the other player or to "defect" against him, which symbolizes betrayal and exploitation. In each round of the game, a player chooses without knowing what his enemy plans to do. If player A defects and player B cooperates, A gets five points and B ends up with a sucker's zero. If both players cooperate, both get three points. If both defect, both end up with a single point.

Sounds like the most competitive, aggressive player wins, right? Here's the catch. Axelrod found that nice guys tend to finish first. He held a worldwide tournament in which he asked people to submit strategies for the game that they thought would win. He used computer technology to pit all the strategies against one another for a thousand games.

The rule for success? A strategy called Tit for Tat. It was one of the simplest strategies submitted, and it went as follows: Always cooperate on your first move. After that, do whatever your opponent did on his previous move. If he cooperated, cooperate. If he defected, hit him back with a swift defection, but then forgive him and be ready to cooperate again.

The successful player doesn't fret and fume or nurse a never-ending grudge. He isn't so nice that he's a sucker; neither does he get involved in a cycle of mutual punishment. He doesn't try to second-guess his enemies. Tit for Tat succeeds—and it's simple, strong and yet forgiving. Most important, it takes the long view and plays for long-term advantage.

much better do you feel? The answer, of course, is: not much. The four remaining tacks are still digging into your flesh. Often you must change many areas of your life in order to be truly vital and energetic.

It is possible. Some of the patients who have surprised me the most are recovering addicts—people who once had absolutely no balance in their life but were on a self-destruct program. These people, on the road to recovery in the health-conscious nineties, can become extremely healthy, adopting a lifestyle that focuses on a "benign" obsession with exercise, good diet, and stress reduction, as well as finding a spiritual community, friends, and families. These are often people who peak in their forties, fifties, and sixties, achieving high degrees of energy they never anticipated would be possible while they were drinking and drugging in their twenties and thirties. The key to their energy is a hard-won wisdom that comes with living and, yes, aging. Aging is not always accompanied by inevitable decline.

Consider this book, then, your strategy for living life as an art.

AFTERWORD

▼

This is a book about combating and curing one of the most common, debilitating, and mysterious ailments of humankind: fatigue. It is about the intricate web of mind and body, immune system and brain, hormones and well-being, environment and genetics. It's about clearing poisons out of your body. It's about allergies, diet, digestion. Above all, it is about getting well.

It is not, however, a book about major illnesses, and so pause here with me to consider something important. Fatigue *is* sometimes a prelude to serious illness. It can be an early-warning sign, and if you listen to it, it can save your life. A study on men who had heart attacks found that a month or two before their illness, they'd experienced vague and debilitating fatigue. Similarly, if you ask cancer patients how they felt in the year before their diagnosis, they'll often admit that things didn't "seem right." They didn't have their usual energy.

I had a patient only recently who came in complaining of fatigue. He was a manager in a machine shop. I checked his pulse and found it wildly irregular. His cholesterol, when last checked, had been in the high 300s. I questioned him extensively, but his answers were brief and unenlightening. Finally I ran an EKG and found that his heart rhythm was erratic. That was when he thumped on his chest and said, "By the way, I'm getting pressure in my heart and it hurts me. I never thought it was a real problem." The truth, as confirmed later by a cardiologist to whom I referred him, was that he was on the verge of a major heart attack.

I find that some people, particularly men, don't go to doctors until they have extremely serious symptoms. Indeed, as a segment on the television news program "20-20" reported, men tend to favor stoicism and denial. Women are far more likely to see doctors, but men will sometimes trudge on, sick almost unto death, before they finally visit their doctor for a dire problem like metastatic lung cancer or crushing chest pain.

There are also some patients whose families have a history of a certain disease, and they are so frightened of it that they avoid ever mentioning it, much less visiting a doctor to determine their risk and, if necessary, change their lifestyle. Someone whose mother has died of sudden cerebral aneurysm (a burst blood vessel in the brain) at age fifty may become terrified by the appearance of ordinary headaches, yet suffer through them silently because he is afraid a doctor may tell him he's at risk for stroke. So often, if patients visited a physician and discussed these fears, they would be relieved to find nothing is wrong— and that dietary and lifestyle changes can help protect them in the future.

If you have been experiencing persistent fatigue, the first action you should take is to make an appointment with your family physician. Most fatigue is *not* due to a major illness, but it is important to have a physician's "all clear" before you follow the approaches recommended in this book. A doctor will perform a checklist of important tests, based on your history, to rule out major illness.

REFERENCES

▼

BOOKS

Benson, Herbert. *The Relaxation Response.* New York: Avon Books, 1976.

Brighthope, Ian, M.D. *Fighting Fatigue and the Chronic Fatigue Syndrome.* Sydney, Australia: McCulloch Publishing, 1990.

Epstein, Gerald, M.D. *Healing Visualizations: Creating Health Through Imagery.* New York: Bantam Books, 1989.

Fixx, James F. *The Complete Book of Running.* New York: Random House, 1977.

Goldberg, Myron D., M. D., and Julie Rubin. *The Inside Tract: Understanding and Preventing Digestive Disorders.* AARP Books, 1986.

Greenberg, Kurt, ed. *Challenging Orthodoxy: America's Top Medical Preventives Speak Out!* New Canaan, CT: Keats Publishing, 1991.

Hamner, Daniel, M.D., and Barbara Burr. *Peak Energy: The High-Oxygen Program for More Energy Now!* New York: Putnam, 1988.

LeShan, Lawrence. *How to Meditate: The Acclaimed Guide to Self-Discovery.* New York: Bantam New Age Books, 1988.

Lewinsohn, Peter M., Ph.D., Ricardo F. Munoz, Ph.D., Mary Ann Youngren, Ph.D., and Antonette M. Zeiss, Ph.D. *Control Your Depression.* New York: Prentice Hall Press, 1986.

Murray, Michael, N.D., and Joseph Pizzorno, N.D. *The Encyclopedia of Natural Medicine.* Rocklin, CA: Prima Publishing, 1991.

Pearsall, Paul, Ph.D. *Making Miracles: A Scientist's Journey to Death and Back Reveals the Powerful Hidden Order Behind Life's Chaos, Crises and Coincidences.* New York: Prentice Hall Press, 1991.

Podell, Richard N., M.D., F.A.C.P. *Doctor, Why Am I So Tired?* New York: Fawcett, 1987.

Randolph, Theron G., M.D., and Ralph W. Moss, Ph.D. *An Alternative Approach to Allergies: The New Field of Clinical Ecology Unravels the En-*

References

vironmental Causes of Mental and Physical Ills. New York: Harper & Row, 1980.

Regestein, Quentin, M.D. *Sleep: Problems and Solutions*. New York: Consumer Reports Books, 1990.

Rogers, Sherry A., M.D. *Tired or Toxic?: A Blueprint for Health*. Syracuse, NY: Prestige Publishers, 1990.

Shorter, Edward. *From Paralysis to Fatigue: A History of Psychosomatic Illness in the Modern Era*. New York: Free Press, 1992.

Singer, Raymond M. *Neurotoxicity Guidebook*. New York: Van Nostrand Reinhold, 1990.

Solomon, Neil, M.D., Ph.D., and Marc Lipton, Ph.D., M.P.A. *Sick and Tired of Being Sick and Tired*. New York: Wynwood Press, 1989.

Truss, C. Orian, M.D. *The Missing Diagnosis*. Truss Books, 1982.

Wurtman, Richard, Michael Baum, and John Potts, Jr., eds. *The Medical and Biological Effects of Light*. Annals of the New York Academy of Sciences, vol. 453.

ARTICLES

Thyroid

Ehrenkranz, Joel R. L., M.D. "Body Temperature Changes: Clues to Endocrine Disease." *Medical Aspects of Human Sexuality*, July 1986, pp. 102–8.

Mu, Lt., and colleagues, "Endemic Goitre in Central China Caused by Excessive Iodine Intake." *The Lancet*, Aug. 1, 1987, p. 257.

Sawin, Clark T., M.D., and Maria H. London, M.D. "Natural Desiccated Thyroid: A Health-Food Thyroid Preparation." *Archives of Internal Medicine* 149 (September 1989).

Tintera, John W., M.D. "The Hypoadrenocortical State and Its Management." *Journal of the American Quack Association* 3, no. 2 (December 1987): 3–7.

Premenstrual Syndrome

Abraham, Guy E., M.D. "Nutritional Factors in the Etiology of the Premenstrual Tension Syndromes." *The Journal of Reproductive Medicine* 18, no. 7 (July 1983).

Goei, Gordon S., M.D., and Guy E. Abraham, M.D. "Effect of a Nutritional Supplement, Optivite, on Symptoms of Premenstrual Tension." *The Journal of Reproductive Medicine* 28, no. 8 (August 1983).

References

Helms, Joseph, M.D. "Acupuncture for the Management of Primary Dysmenorrhea." *Obstetrics and Gynecology* 69, no. 1 (January 1987).

"Premenstrual Syndrome May Be Entirely Due to Thyroid Disease." *Internal Medicine News* 19, no. 12, p. 43.

"Thyroid Hypofunction in Premenstrual Syndrome." *The New England Journal of Medicine*, Dec. 4, 1986, p. 1486.

Fatigue

Kroenke, Kurt, M.D. "Symptoms in Medical Patients: An Untended Field." *The American Journal of Medicine* 92 (Jan. 24, 1992), pp. 1A–3S.

Leskowitc, Eric. "Life Energy and Western Medicine: A Reappraisal." *Advances* 8, no. 1 (Winter 1992): 63.

Sugar Disease

Crapo, Phyllis A., R.D. "Theory vs. Fact: The Glycemic Response to Foods." *Nutrition Today*, March/April 1984, pp. 6–11.

"Evaluation of Health Aspects of Sugars Contained in Carbohydrate Sweeteners," Report of Sugars Task Force, 1986, *The Journal of Clinical Nutrition* 116, no. 11S (November 1986). Supplement.

Field, James, M.D. "Catch a Falling Sugar." *Emergency Medicine*, Nov. 30, 1985, pp. 19–36.

Fredericks, Carlton. *Low Blood Sugar and You*. New York: Grosset & Dunlap, 1969.

"Hypertension, Lipids and Cardiovascular Disease: Is Insulin the Missing Link?" Proceedings of a Symposium. *The American Journal of Medicine* 90 (Feb. 21, 1991).

Reaven, Gerald. "Role of Insulin Resistance in Human Disease," *Diabetes* 37 (December 1988).

Walker, Arp, D.Sc. "Sugar: A Love/Hate Situation." *International Clinical Nutrition Review* 11, no. 1 (January 1991): 10–23.

Wolever, Thomas M. S., et al. "The Glycemic Index: Methodology and Clinical Implications." *American Journal of Clinical Nutrition* 54 (1991): 846–54.

Wurtman, Judith, Ph.D. "Carbohydrate Craving, Mood Changes, and Obesity." *Health Media of America* 5, no. 10 (October 1987).

Environmental Toxins

Aposhian, H. Vasken. "DMSA and DMPS—Water Soluble Antidotes for Heavy Metal Poisoning." *Annual Review of Pharmacological Toxicology* 23 (1983): 193–215.

References

"Beverages Intoxicated by Lead in Crystal." *Science News* 139, no. 4 (Jan. 26, 1991).

Buchet, J. P., et al. "Renal Effects of Cadmium Body Burden of the General Population." *The Lancet* 336: 669–702.

"Eliminating the Lead in Your Tap Water." *Wellness Letter*, University of California at Berkeley, April 1987.

Mahaffey, Kathryn R., Ph.D., et al. "National Estimates of Blood Lead Levels: United States, 1976–1980." *The New England Journal of Medicine* 307, no. 10 (Sept. 2, 1982).

"Mercury in Pituitary Glands of Dentists," *The Lancet*, February 22, 1986, p. 442.

"Office Buildings That Breathe." *The New York Times*, Feb. 9, 1992, p. 9.

Reinhold, Robert. "When Life Is Toxic." *The New York Times Magazine*, Sept. 16, 1990, pp. 50–70.

Terr, Abba, M.D. "Environmental Illness: A Clinical Review of 50 Cases." *Archives of Internal Medicine* 146 (January 1986): 145–52.

Wedeen, Richard P., M.D. "Low-Level Lead Poisoning in Adults." *Drug Therapy*, September 1986, pp. 78–85.

Sleep

"Caffeine Jitters." *FDA Consumer*, December 1987/January 1988, pp. 22–27.

Canter, Mark, "Are You Light-Starved?" *Yoga Journal*, July/August 1988.

"Disturbances in Sleep Rhythm: Jet Lag." *International Clinical Nutrition Review* 7, no. 2 (April 1987): 78.

Krupp, Lauren, and Wallace Mendelson, M.D. "Sleep Disorders in Chronic Fatigue Syndrome." *Sleep*, Pontenagel Press, Bochum, 1990, pp. 261–63.

"The Use of Light for Health and Healing." *Healthfacts*, Center for Medical Consumers, vol. 11, no. 81 (February 1986).

Exercise and Nutrition

Davis, J. Mark, Ph.D., et al. "Carbohydrate-Electrolyte Drinks: Effects on Endurance Cycling in the Heat." *American Journal of Clinical Nutrition* 48 (1988): 1023–30.

Keen, Carl, Ph.D. "Trace Elements in Athletic Performance," *Sport, Health and Nutrition*, vol. 2, from *The 1984 Olympic Scientific Congress Proceedings*.

Kleiner, Susan, Ph.D. "Performance-Enhancing Aids in Sport." *Journal of the American College of Nutrition* 10 (1991): 163–76.

McNaughton, Lars, Ph.D. "A Review of Some Nutritional Ergogonic Aids." *International Clinical Nutrition Review* 6, no. 2 (April 1986), pp. 70–87.

Schwartz, Tony. "Making Waves: Can Dr. Irv Dardik's Radical Exercise Therapy Really Work Miracles?" *New York*, Mar. 18, 1991, pp. 31–39.

References

Depression

Dullea, Georgia. "Winter Depression: Shedding Light on Dark-Day Blues." *The New York Times*, Dec. 19, 1985, p. C1.

Nesse, Randolph. "What Good Is Feeling Bad?" *The Sciences*, November/December 1991, pp. 30–37.

Schleifer, Steven, M.D. "Altered Lymphocyte Function in the Depressed Patient." *Infections in Medicine*, April 1991, pp. 42–46.

Silver, Nan. "Do Optimists Live Longer?" *American Health*, November 1986, pp. 50–53.

Molds

"Damp, Moldy Housing and Health." *Journal Watch*, Aug. 1, 1989, p. 19.

Rogers, Sherry, M.D. "The Many Guises of Mold Allergy." *Bestways Magazine*, January 1986.

Chronic Fatigue Syndrome

Bankhead, Charles. "Fibromyalgia May Really Be in the Muscle, Not the Mind." *Medical World News*, Sept. 12, 1988.

"CFIDS Research Vaults Forward." The CFIDS Chronicle, *Journal of the Chronic Fatigue and Immune Dysfunction Syndrome Association*, Fall 1991.

"Chronic Fatigue: Epstein-Barr Connection Disputed." *Medical World News*, June 13, 1988, p. 35.

Jamal, Goran, and Stig Hansen. "Post-Viral Fatigue Syndrome." The Glasgow University Department of Neurology, *European Neurology* 29 (1989): 273–76.

Kroenke, Kurt, M.D. "Chronic Fatigue in Primary Care." *Journal of the American Medical Association* 260, no. 7 (Aug. 19, 1988): 929–34.

Landay, Alan, et al. "Chronic Fatigue Syndrome: Clinical Condition Associated with Immune Activation." *The Lancet* 339, no. 8769 (Sept. 21, 1991): 707–11.

Latman, Lawrence, "Virus Found That May Be Linked to a Debilitating Fatigue Ailment." *New York Times*, Sept. 5, 1990.

"Several Abnormalities Linked with Fatigue Syndrome." *Internal Medicine News*, vol. 21, no. 4, p. 23.

Straus, Stephen, M.D. "Intravenous Immunoglobulin Treatment for the Chronic Fatigue Syndrome." *The American Journal of Medicine* 89 (November 1990): 551–68.

"Successful Treatment of Chronic Active Epstein-Barr Virus Infection with Recombinant Interleukin-2." *The Lancet*, Jan. 17, 1987, p. 154.

"Treatment of Lyme Disease." *The Medical Letter on Drugs and Therapeutics* 31, issue 794 (June 16, 1989).

INDEX

▼